CHRONIC

CHRONIC
UNDERSTANDING PAIN

GILLIAN BEST

ICON

Published in the UK in 2026 by
Icon Books Ltd, Omnibus Business Centre,
39–41 North Road, London N7 9DP
email: info@iconbooks.com
www.iconbooks.com

ISBN: 978-183773-272-2
ebook: 978-183773-274-6

Typesetting by SJmagic DESIGN SERVICES, India

Printed and bound in the UK

Appointed GPSR EU Representative: Easy Access System Europe Oü, 16879218
Address: Mustamäe tee 50, 10621, Tallinn, Estonia
Contact Details: gpsr.requests@easproject.com, +358 40 500 3575

For Kerri

CONTENTS

Prologue ix

1 Pain, the basics 1
2 Can CAR T-cell therapy treat my disease(s)? 17
3 Your brain is in pain 27
4 Sex differences in pain 87
5 What's the central nervous system got to do with it? 111
6 The beginning, genetically speaking 133
7 Did I get this from my parents? 159
8 How your perception of your body alters your pain experience 167
9 Predicting pain 177
10 Chronic pain on a population-wide level 187
11 How to improve chronic pain research 217
12 What if pain isn't driven by the brain? 227
13 Stopping inflammation and repairing it too 243

The end 253
Acknowledgements 261
Index 263

PROLOGUE

I'm writing this from the hospital. It's cold and brightly lit. My nurse today, a lovely woman named Jolly, is frowning at the cannula because I won't bleed for her. It's nothing personal, I'm just not a great bleeder. I can feel her try to shimmy the needle into my vein a bit more; something about seeing her do that makes it hurt, or maybe that's just what I think, so I look away. What I do know is that we need to get three vials of blood and so far we've got maybe half of one. Jolly gets the bright blue elastic band and together we tie it on my arm, just above the elbow. We leave it there for a moment and then untie it, both of us watching and hoping the vial will fill. No such luck. She massages the vein, which doesn't work, so we move my arm off the arm rest and see if gravity might help. It doesn't. I apologise profusely for the stubbornness of my blood. We decide to cut our losses and try after my infusion is done.

Every eight weeks I drag myself here, where I'm greeted like an old friend by the nurses who welcome me into the biologics day unit. I'm assigned a chair that's more like a bed, and someone weighs me and puts a cannula into my arm. Blood pressure, heart rate, and temperature are all checked before they hang the drip bag that contains my medicine.

I'll sit here for the next hour and a half, while it slowly drips into me, delivering something called Tumour Necrosis Factor alpha blocker (or TNF) that's meant to suppress my arthritis. I think of it as a Xanax for my immune system, which really needs to chill out. I've been coming here every eight weeks since May 2023, when I came for my first of three loading doses – this was after most of the other biologics I could try didn't work for me and my main diseases, which are ankylosing spondylitis (AS) and Crohn's disease.

AS is an inflammatory autoimmune arthritis that causes my spine and hips to do their best to fuse. It is, quite literally, a pain in the ass. That's how it first presented for me: a pain so excruciating in my sitting bones that I couldn't get out of bed to go to the bathroom. When I was eighteen, my brother brought me his skateboard and wheeled me down the hall to the toilet, so I narrowly escaped having an accident.

Doctors call AS a 'complex condition', which means that it's an overachiever when it comes to symptoms and other related issues. You can have Crohn's disease with it (like I do), a really miserable eye disease called uveitis, where your eye can go really red and inflamed (and which can, in some cases, make you go blind) or your pupil takes over your whole eye, which then starts leaking. Any light – even the dullest – feels like a thousand hot knives stabbing at your eye. This form of arthritis can also give you excruciating pain in your ribs or chest (I get this, it's absolutely horrendous). It feels like a heart attack. It's called costochondritis, this inflammation of your rib joints. Anyhow, you get the picture: AS is not a disease you want to get.

One in every two hundred people in the UK have this form of arthritis, which is twice as many as multiple sclerosis and Parkinson's disease. On the McGill Pain Index,[1] it's right up there with childbirth and kidney stones.

I've had kidney stones and can confirm: that's a very accurate pain scale. (And at least the kidney stones go away eventually. AS is with you for life.) Even though I'm not in agony every day, my pain is significant enough to take biologics, which I started trying about five years ago. Most of those medications are available in the self-stab epi-pen format, but not the one that works for me. And that's why I'm here at the biologics day unit.

There are eight beds in this unit, where people stay for as little as thirty minutes and as long as five hours. In the middle of the room are a couple of stands, one has a laptop, the other has masks and biscuits. Beside that are two disposal bins. The soundtrack is muffled talk and the beeping

---

[1] https://www.burningnightscrps.org/crps/crps-information/what-is-crps/

of drip machines. I seem to run afoul of my machine pretty often – it complains by beeping loudly whenever I bend my arm too much. A nurse will come over and tut gently at me, straighten out my arm, and remind me that I have to not bend so much. It's not like I'm doing yoga, I'm just tapping away on my laptop, but there's no pleasing these machines some days. While I'm here, the machine and I are tethered together – it's my ball and chain. It comes to the bathroom with me, which can be tricky: the drip rack handles about as well as a supermarket trolley.

For now, the treatment works well enough for me to keep taking it, which is good because some (just some!) of the side effects are diseases that don't come with happy endings. The side effects can range from the banal (headache, nausea), to the concerning (heart failure), to the deeply worrying (malignancy – half of the cases reported are lymphomas).

When you're willing to take your chances with cancer, you know your pain is bad.

I'd rather not take this drug, or any of the other drugs that are meant to treat my disease. Even the milder side effects aren't fun. Long-term use of a type of drug called NSAIDs (non-steroidal anti-inflammatories, things like Aspirin, Naproxen) have given me tinnitus. A drug that used to work really well for me, called Vioxx, was taken off the market because people kept having heart attacks.

There are times when the pain is so bad that I need what I like to call my 'Big Girl' painkillers. Things like kidney-stone grade codeine, tramadol, or a nice anti-spasmodic like baclofen (because when you've been holding yourself in a twisted, contorted posture for days on end, hoping this flare will pass, you can't just relax out of it). Getting the painkillers I need when I'm in excruciating pain is no small feat – more than once I've been asked if I'm 'drug-seeking'. I've been given, begrudgingly, the most meagre prescription for something that never really takes the edge fully off. 'Have you tried paracetamol? A hot bath?' That's not bad advice, but when I'm crying because I'm in so much pain, and exhausted because I haven't slept due to the pain, and can't really eat because of the pain …

It's not like these drugs really do the trick either. Usually, they just make me care less about the fact that, for instance, my neck doesn't feel strong enough to hold my head up and I can't move it to the left or right or up or down. Other times, maybe they'll knock me out enough so I can sleep when my ribs hurt so much it feels like I can't breathe, sit, stand, lie down or move around.

I'm grateful to the kind nurses and doctors who treat me, and I'm grateful to the researchers who developed the medication I take because it really is a game-changer. But I don't want to go to the hospital all the time. I don't want to worry about scary side effects. I don't want to be sick anymore. I don't want to think about my body and the ways in which it's dysfunctional, broken or just plain hurts. I'm tired of designing my days around keeping my body functioning. It's exhausting. The treatment that works today could stop tomorrow – or I could be taken off it because the side effects become intolerable.

I've spent more of my life in pain than not, and what I really want is a cure. There's a chance that a new treatment some researchers in Germany have developed which has CURED people with a disease sort of similar to mine might work, but it's a long shot. I'll need to find a cellular target, and to do that I'm going to need to talk to some really clever researchers. But just in case I can't find a cure, I'll happily settle for some answers. I want to know where pain comes from. Why don't our existing drugs treat it very well? Where are the new drugs? What are the next treatments for chronic pain? Who's working on this stuff? What are they doing?

To find out, I'm going to talk to the world-leading researchers and scientists working in chronic pain, rheumatology, genetics, immunology and psychiatry so that I can understand pain – what it is, where it comes from – and, importantly, how to get rid of it. I want to understand what we're doing now, and what the future could hold.

This book is about my quest to understand my true enemy – chronic pain. Getting to the bottom of questions I've had for years. At the very least I'll get a better understanding of how chronic pain works, and how we might one day get rid of it. What have I got to lose?

Certainly not a lot of blood. Back in the biologics unit, my infusion is finished. Jolly comes over after her lunch break and we try again. She presses the vial into the cannula and we go through the process once more. She massages the vein. I tell her I've spent my infusion drinking a ton of water. She tells me it's not my fault. And then, finally, the blood starts to sort of, reluctantly, drip out. We get enough to run their tests, the cannula is removed, and the drip stand and I part ways. I'm free to go about my life for the next eight weeks, until I'm back and we go through the whole thing again.

PAIN, THE BASICS 1

'Pain is so fundamental, it's hard-wired into us and all other animals. It gets overlooked in medicine because people go for the disease. And yet what takes people to ask for help is often the pain. I'm not saying we shouldn't treat disease, of course we should and if the pain goes away, that's great. But too often it doesn't.'

Amanda Williams, Professor of Clinical Health Psychology, UCL

Chronic pain. If you've got it, I feel for you.

We're not alone: it's estimated that 1.5 billion people live with chronic pain around the world.[1] That's a lot of people in a lot of pain.

I type pain into Google and some related searches include symptoms, treatment and examples, but my favourite has to be: is life worth living with chronic pain? I'd argue that

[1] https://www.nature.com/articles/s41598-023-49761-3

when you've got chronic pain, what you call life and living are different. I'll put my hand up here and say that I don't have it as bad as some people. I know other people have it so much worse – I'm not immobilised, I'm able to hold down a full-time day job and generally make my life work. I'm also lucky enough to have a very supportive partner, family and employer. I have everything necessary to function as well as possible.

I also have a well-stocked pharmacy at home, a smaller travelling pharmacy, and a heating pad in almost every room of my house (because who wants to fiddle around with a plug behind the couch when it hurts to move?).

But what exactly is chronic pain? Traditionally, we're taught that it's any pain that lasts longer than three months. That's what the NHS will tell you. But it's not just that. If you're suffering from chronic pain you know it's so much more than that – it's your life. We need a definition that represents how we feel and what we go through, and one with enough room in it for everyone's pain, so we can get the treatment we need.

Amanda Williams, Professor of Clinical Health Psychology at University College London (UCL), has proposed (along with her colleague Kenneth Craig) a more expansive definition of pain. In their paper they write: 'A definition needs to work for clinical and experimental pain, for humans and for other animals, for excruciating and for trivial pain. It needs to distinguish pain from all other sources of distress, from specific anxieties to existential angst or profound grief.'

They were asked to suggest a new definition for chronic pain, but were reluctant because they thought it should be for a multidisciplinary group to develop, as it had been before. But what they did provide was this: 'Pain is a distressing experience associated with actual or potential tissue damage with sensory, emotional, cognitive, and social components.' Professor Williams tells me that, 'What is important, I think, is that for humans there should be cognitive and social components alongside the sensory and emotional components.'[2]

There's a lot of room in that definition and that's good because it needs to cover a wide variety of things. And when we take all that and add time to make it chronic, it makes it easier to believe everyone who says they're in pain. Not that belief is a cure in and of itself (more on that later), but it's a good start.

There's a shift happening in the way we think about pain and that affects how it's treated. Previously, doctors might have focused on treating your chronic pain at the site where it hurts, but now we're seeing a move towards introducing psychology to ease its impact.

Before we go any further, it's really important to highlight that using psychology does not mean that people aren't in physical pain. All the researchers I spoke with for this book went to great lengths to say – sometimes over and over again – how much they believe people who say they're in pain and how much this isn't about it being made up.

---

[2] https://www.iasp-pain.org/publications/relief-news/article/definition-pain/

The thing is that our brains are really strong – and this approach is working. I don't know about you, but if there's a way to ease my pain that actually works, I'm here for that.

There are three flavours of pain, and they all suck. Obviously. But it's important to have these classifications for a lot of different reasons, the main one being treatment. If you don't know what the problem is, you can't treat it. And even in the sometimes murky world of chronic pain and confusing symptoms, there are three main classifications that are helpful.

The first is the kind of pain we've all experienced from time to time, the sharp, achy throbbing kind. The run of the mill, stubbed your toe or having a dental procedure kind of pain. That's called **nociceptive pain**. The International Association for the Study of Pain (IASP) describes it as: pain that arises from actual or threatened damage to non-neural tissue and is due to the activation of nociceptors.

It's the non-neural tissue that I want to highlight to you here. Not brain stuff is what it boils down to. What are nociceptors? The IASP says: 'A high-threshold sensory receptor of the peripheral somatosensory nervous system that is capable of transducing and encoding noxious stimuli.' Or, a part of your nervous system that can turn damage into pain.

The second pain features numbness, tingling and weakness in your hands, arms or feet. That's **neuropathic pain** and it's caused by damage to a part of the somatosensory nervous system. The most common cause? In the UK, it's nerve damage from diabetes. Neuropathic pain is nerve pain that happens if your nervous system messes up or gets damaged. You can experience pain from any of the various levels of your nervous system, and those levels include your peripheral nerves, your spinal cord and your brain – which when taken together form your central nervous system, or CNS for short.

And the last kind is one that maybe you've heard your doctors talking about, called **nociplastic pain** (pronounced no-see-plastic), and you get it a lot in in fibromyalgia, headaches and low back pain. This type of pain is different from nociceptive pain in the way it produces symptoms. We don't really know what causes this third wheel of pain, but researchers and doctors reckon that 'augmented central nervous system pain' and 'sensory processing and altered pain modulation' play prominent roles. The short version is that this is the pain that lives in your brain.

Symptoms here include pain that's more widespread or intense – or both! – and includes things like fatigue, sleep, memory, and mood problems (like depression). This type of pain can occur in isolation, as often happens with fibromyalgia or tension headaches, or with ongoing nociceptive or neuropathic pain. A classic example here is chronic low back pain.

The *Lancet*, an important and influential medical journal aimed at doctors, helpfully adds that, 'It is important to recognise this type of pain,' and part of me feels like we should put that on a banner in the GP's office. The article goes on to say that treatments for other kinds of pain aren't going to work very well on this type.[3]

---

[3] https://www.thelancet.com/journals/lancet/article/PIIS0140-6736(21)00392-5/abstract

The first time nociplastic pain was mentioned in a scientific paper was in 2016, and there is still some controversy around it – mostly that its name is misleading and that it may not exist as an autonomous phenomenon. This type of pain 'arises from actual or threatened damage to non-neural tissue and is due to the activation of nociceptors', which are 'high-threshold sensory receptors of the peripheral somatosensory nervous system that are capable of transducing and encoding noxious stimuli'.[4] So it's pain that happens when tissue outside the brain perceives or experiences damage and nociceptors get switched on.

As to where this type of pain comes from, the most likely triggers – things that might predispose you to it – include a history of abuse, environmental exposure and genetics. Oh – and this won't be surprising if you're a woman – studies show that in female mice, it's easier to induce this kind of pain than in male mice. The importance of the neuropathic/nociceptive distinction is that if we're talking about drug treatments, drugs that treat one don't touch the other, and vice versa.

The vocabulary we have to describe pain is also really important. Traditional options include: burning, sharp, stabbing, throbbing, cramping, aching, radiating, dull and shooting. But it feels like chronic pain deserves something more, especially when you consider that one third of the world's population is in pain every day.[6]

---

[4] https://www.iasp-pain.org/resources/terminology/

When I speak with Professor Simon Beggs, Associate Professor, Developmental Neurosciences Department, at UCL's Great Ormond Street Institute of Child Health, he reminds me of something that's obvious if you've ever tried to describe chronic pain to a doctor – it's really tricky to accurately convey. 'It's not well described. The biggest cause of sick days is lumbar back pain. And people say, oh, I've had that. It's all right. You just get moving and you're fine. And that's not the same as someone who's got crippling arthritis. But it's all the same word that describes it. Because everyone has an experience of pain, so they think everyone else's experience is the same,' he says. 'Chronic pain is devastating.'

He's not wrong. When you're telling someone – a friend, family member or co-worker – about your pain and they say, 'Oh, I've had a bad back, here's what I did,' as Professor Beggs says, those helpful suggestions will be so woefully inadequate as to feel insulting. Pain is such a personal, individual experience that it's difficult to get across the idea that some pain is different than others. But pain isn't a competition. This is what my sister (who has the same disease I do) and I are always trying to explain to our mother when her 80-year-old back aches. Everyone can be in pain, everyone can hurt. That's valid. But for some people it's so much worse.

But if we don't tell doctors about our pain, they can't try to treat it. Before each rheumatologist appointment I fill in eight questionnaires, providing my specialist Professor Raj Sengupta with a picture of what my disease activity has been like over the week preceding the appointment. Disease activity seems like a fairly weak euphemism for pain, but some people can have a lot of disease activity and no pain.

Questionnaires may seem lo-fi or woefully inadequate, but how else can we measure pain? Remember the definition that Professor Williams had – pain is an emotional experience. Even if we could measure pain in a really simple and straightforward way, how you experience it and how I experience it are going to be different because we're different people.

But why do we even have to measure it in the first place? Doctors have to be able to measure it so they can treat it. Medicine is numbers-based. Your pain is a six out of ten, the doctor gives you a tablet, you check back in a few weeks later and the pain is a three. So the tablet works. When I started my infusions, we took a baseline of my pain, which over a week was something like a six. After about three months of infusions, I did my pain scores again, and they were much lower, so we could say that the infusions were working.

It's difficult to put into words the vastness, the sheer enormity, of chronic pain and the strange world it can plunge or drag you into. The days where you're too ill to work and sort of drift around in agony, thinking about your pain, trying everything and anything you can think of to ease it, and when that fails, doing your utmost to bear it. Time moves differently on those days; it's slow and foggy. It's a solitary state in which you exist, a miserable sort of limbo where you're constantly braced: waiting for things to get better or worse. I remind myself when I'm in this state that it won't last, that things will get different. I never say better, that feels dangerous, like I'm setting myself up for the kind of disappointment that's difficult to get over. There's not much else you can do in this state but live through it. You endure pain, you ride it out.

Of course, it's not just you who has to somehow cope with this; it's everyone who knows and loves you. I wonder sometimes which is worse: suffering through it yourself, or having to watch someone else go through it, knowing there's no way to help. They can be there for you, listen to you, help with chores and life admin, but that never feels like enough. Or rather, that's not how they want to help. They want to take the burden of living with pain away, but they can't.

Sometime early on in my relationship with my partner, I had a flare. A band of super-deep low pressure flung itself across the UK – low pressure is often a trigger for me – and sure enough, my AS flared. It was the first time my partner had ever experienced me in a flare, wincing with every movement. My mom sent him an email – a sort of introductory email, I guess. About what it was like caring for me when I was going through a flare. She always talks of a particular facial expression I have when I'm really suffering – for her, that's the telltale sign that this is Really Bad.

But not all days are like this. There are better ones, and when you get a string of them, and they turn into months and even years that are only punctuated by a few bad days, you get to a point where you feel almost normal. You do your exercises, take your vitamins, get enough sleep, and somehow the pain stays away.

Until it comes back. It always does.

This is almost always followed by a well-meaning question from a person with good intentions who is genuinely surprised that your pain is back. Why is this happening to you? What have you done? When someone asks this question it can feel like you're being blamed. As in, you were doing well there, why'd you let yourself fall off the pain-free wagon?

As though it were a personal decision. As though any rational human who is very familiar with the limits of pain-killing drugs available would ever willingly put themselves in a position to experience pain again. It's not like we miss it.

If you confess you don't really know why the pain's back, that seems to provide, for some people, an opening to speculate. They'll list off reasons why their grandmother's arthritis flares up, which segues into helpful suggestions of how to alleviate the pain, and that almost always includes things like apple cider vinegar and chilli peppers. At no point in time are these helpful souls interested in hearing about the fact that medical science hasn't quite worked it all out yet.

There's fear behind the question, a worry that if the world really is random enough for me to be in this much pain for no good reason, then what's stopping it from attacking them? They're afraid of this random stroke of bad luck. It's important for there to be an answer to why my disease is behaving like this, right now. People who are outside the day-to-day living with chronic pain need to believe that cause and effect is a fact.

I know the answer is that I have ankylosing spondylitis. That's why my body hurts so much. This is not a good answer.

'Yes, but why? You were fine yesterday.'

I almost certainly wasn't, but probably the pain was manageable and so I didn't bother mentioning it. Even with the people who love you the most, there's always that feeling, and sometimes it's just a twinge, other times it's quite sharp, that they will run out of patience listening to you. It's exhausting, chronic pain and chronic illness. You can't go through life expecting people to listen every morning as you reel off a list of body parts that hurt. They find it exasperating, and after a while they can't take it anymore.

The grinding monotony of chronic pain and chronic disease are really the hardest parts to bear. It's the consistency of it that catches people by surprise. Maybe it's because sometimes there are days and weeks even, when the pain isn't intolerable and you can look and act like a Normal Person. That can trick anyone into thinking that things are better, that the pain is gone. The truth of the matter is that I don't know, and the doctors don't either. Maybe it's just that, after having this disease for so long, I've become used to the unpredictability of it. Sometimes there's a reason for a flare – a long-haul flight is never easy, or if my schedule is too packed and I don't get enough time in the pool or out walking – but it doesn't have to be those things. You never really know. And I suppose if you don't have to get used to that, it's hard to understand why anyone would.

But what if there was a chance to develop a cure?

On 15 September 2022, the *Guardian* published an article called 'Scientists hail autoimmune disease therapy breakthrough'.[5] The standfirst read: 'Study finds CAR T-cell treatment sends lupus into remission, raising hopes it could be used to treat ...'

In CAR T therapy, T cells – part of our immune system that normally kills infected cells – are taken from a person's blood sample, grown in the laboratory and 're-programmed' to recognise and kill cancer cells just as they would naturally attack an infected cell. The reprogramming is done by introducing a gene for an artificial protein called a chimeric antigen receptor, or CAR for short. It's used to treat rare, incurable cancers such as leukaemia, lymphoma and multiple myeloma.

It was the very last line of the article that sent my mind into overdrive: 'Several other autoimmune diseases ... these include rheumatoid arthritis ...'

After reading the article, I could feel my hope coming back. I decided that I'd try to engineer a situation where I could be involved in a clinical trial of my own. That's not quite as far-fetched as it sounds: my day job is in UCL's fundraising department, so I've seen how – with a generous donation – clinical trials are started. I've been doing this for over twelve years, and I've become familiar with some of the big-deal areas of medical research, particularly cancer. Which is why I knew what CAR T therapy was when I read that

---

[5] https://www.theguardian.com/science/2022/sep/15/scientists-hail-autoimmune-disease-therapy-breakthrough-car-t-cell-lupus

article: UCL happens to be leading the way in the field for this kind of therapy. In fact, the University holds 117 CAR T related patents.

For the patients in the article I'd read, CAR T therapy had cured their lupus. Full remission. One hundred per cent cured. This therapy had essentially rebooted their immune systems.

Nothing's perfect, though. According to cancer.org, possible CAR T-cell therapy side effects can include: Cytokine release syndrome (CRS). As CAR T-cells multiply, they can release large amounts of chemicals called cytokines into the blood, which can ramp up the immune system. Serious side effects from this release can include fever, trouble breathing, nausea, vomiting, headaches and fast heartbeat. You can also experience nervous system problems, which can include symptoms such as: changes in consciousness, seizures, and trouble speaking and understanding.

My rheumatologist, Professor Raj Sengupta, is a wonderful human being and quick with a smile. He's open-minded, curious and exactly the guy you'd want on your team: a specialist who genuinely listens and treats his patients as equals. When I told him about my idea, he said, 'OK, come to my research day and we'll talk about it.' I went and didn't so much talk with him about it as bombard him with ideas.

This idea of patient involvement in research isn't out of the ordinary. In fact, these days, it's often a requirement to include patients in your research proposal to help guide the work. Why would you want to involve the public and patients in your research?

PPI (patient and public involvement) work across research has developed over the last twenty years from being 'a nice idea to do if possible', to a funding requirement for big name funders. The push has come from researchers and their funders, but also from patients and the public; there is increasing evidence that health research done with PPI gets better outcomes for patients. Why? Because patients get to prioritise research topics that matter most to them. And because patients who live with health problems are often in better positions to know what the unanswered questions are to their condition, and what research would most likely improve their quality of life. Plus, patient input at the very start is more likely to improve recruitment to clinical trials.[6]

Raj agreed to think about my CAR T-cell idea and said he'd check with his research partner who coincidentally also works at UCL. Raj agreed that if this collaborator, Pedro Machado, Professor of Rheumatology and Neuromuscular Diseases, thought the idea had legs then we'd arrange a call and talk about next steps. Great, I thought. Job done. I sat back and made a list of all the fundraisers I knew who might be willing to help me get funding for a clinical trial.

If you're not familiar with clinical trials, let me fill you in. It takes about seventeen years, on average, to get from bench (foundational science idea) to bedside (treatment). And even

[6] https://www.medsci.ox.ac.uk/research/patient-and-public-involvement/section-2-what-is-patient-and-public-involvement/why-involve-the-public-in-research

after you get through a successful clinical trial, it's not like you just snap your fingers and the drug's available.

New drugs usually go through three trial phases: Phase I does basic things like determine if the drug is safe, what are the side effects, and how the drug works in the body. They last between one and six months, and usually include from ten to fifty healthy participants. Phase II trials last between three and eighteen months, have about the same number of participants, and look at things like: how effective is the drug, how much of it should be taken and how often. This phase also looks at safety because the trial is using a larger group of people so uncommon side effects could appear. Phase III trials last from twelve to thirty months, have thirty to a hundred participants, and check out safety, efficacy, and whether there's a risk or benefit to a specific population.

There's a whole bunch of other stuff you have to do to start a clinical trial, things like get ethics approval, recruit patients to test it on, get a sponsor (an entity – usually a university or a pharma company) who will be legally responsible for the trial, a funder, chief investigation officer, national coordinating investigator responsible for each trial site, and a principal investigator (this is the person in charge of the research site).

If you run a trial for a new drug at a university in the UK, it'll cost you on average about £1.2 million. That's just the one phase of your trial. That doesn't include all the years of foundational research that has to be done just to get to that point.

After that's finished, the data from clinical trials are documented in a regulatory filing and submitted to the local relevant regulatory agency. Then the marketing application is reviewed by the local regulatory authority, and then the drug is (hopefully) approved by the local regulatory agency if its benefits outweigh its risks. Then it's made available.

And that's if the drug passes all the trials.

Pedro got back to Raj about my idea of a CAR T clinical trial for AS and the answer was no. The therapy wouldn't work because we didn't have a cellular target to train the CAR T on for ankylosing spondylitis. And that was that. No target, no trial.

But I don't give up easy. I suppose that's one thing I've learned from all these years living with pain: when it hurts, you have to keep moving. If you don't you might just get stuck in that position forever.

CAN CAR T-CELL THERAPY TREAT MY DISEASE(S)? 2

The short answer is no.

University College London Hospital was one of three hospitals in the UK running a trial testing CAR T-cell therapy on lupus – just like the researchers in Germany, led by Georg Schett, that were the focus of that article I'd read in the *Guardian*.

In February 2024, they opened an international Phase I study to learn more about the safety and what the potential side effects were. The trial was the first in the UK to look at the potential of CAR T therapy to treat a disease other than cancer. The patients enrolled in it all had lupus.

What happens in cancer to make the CAR T-cells is that the patient's white blood cells are genetically modified to recognise and attack problem-causing cells, in particular B cells (a type of white blood cell that creates antibodies). In people with lupus, B cells become dysfunctional and produce too many autoantibodies, causing inflammation in healthy tissue. This inflammation is what leads to many lupus symptoms.

When the symptoms and inflammation aren't under control, they can cause organ damage. So the idea of this new therapy is that CAR T could help to get rid of the cells that are causing the problems in the first place, through training the T cells to kill the B cells. Better yet, researchers hope that the one-off CAR T therapy will reduce, or even remove, the need for life-long medication for patients with severe lupus.

That sounds awfully close to a cure, doesn't it?

The first person in the UK to have this treatment is 32-year-old Katherine, who had the therapy administered in Manchester in July 2024. She'd tried all the usual treatments – like steroids and immunosuppressants – and they didn't work for her. She'd been living with constant joint pain, extreme fatigue, inflammation and a weakened immune system.

She told researchers: 'I'd lived a normal life until my late 20s, but getting lupus turned my life upside down. I had to give up my job in banking. I had difficulty just getting out of bed, climbing the stairs and even doing day-to-day tasks. I was forced to adapt to living life in a different way. I cried happy tears going home from that appointment, thinking that there was a chance I could wake up every morning without pain, being able to do things like play with my daughter, and imagining all the possibilities of living a somewhat normal life – it felt amazing.'[1]

---

1 https://www.ucl.ac.uk/news/2024/nov/cancer-therapy-potential-transform-lupus-treatment-delivered-uk-first

And at about six weeks after the treatment, she said: 'Even though I wasn't expecting to feel this better so quickly, I do feel I have more energy and I have had no joint swelling. I'm feeling hopeful for the future.'

It's easy to empathise with Katherine as she moves into this exciting new world where her pain is so much less, and where she gets to enjoy life instead of manage her disease.

Dr Maria Leandro is an investigator on the trial, and is part of UCL's Division of Medicine and a Consultant Rheumatologist at University College London Hospital. When she and I meet to chat about the trial and the potential it holds, she starts by telling me that she came to the UK from Portugal, and when she arrived, she did a PhD with Professor Jonathan Edwards.

This is important because he was instrumental in the discovery of the use of B-cell depletion therapy (rituximab) to treat rheumatoid arthritis. B cells are a type of white blood cell that make infection-fighting antibodies. They're a massively important part of your immune system. Rituximab was developed and licensed originally for lymphoma, but they extended the use to rheumatoid arthritis and lupus. (It's mainly used to treat non-Hodgkin's lymphoma.) The idea was that in rheumatoid arthritis, it was the B cells that were behind the inflammation. B cells can also produce harmful autoantibodies which attack the body's own cells and tissues – this is an autoimmune disorder. If you have an autoimmune disease, you'll be familiar with the symptoms: pain, swollen glands, fatigue, rashes, nausea and so on.

Dr Leandro says, 'The hypothesis is that if you kill B cells, and if you also deplete the antibodies that contributed to the disease, then you could cure the disease.' Initially, researchers used rituximab because it's an antibody that binds to B cells, kind of like painting a target on the backs of the B cells. So, your immune system recognises them as something that needs to be killed and then it kills them. In the work Professor Edwards started the patients they treated responded really well.

New B cells usually come back about six to nine months after treatment. When two of the patients experienced flares, they were treated again with rituximab, and again it worked.

'Rituximab doesn't specify normal or abnormal B cells, and once the treatment effect is over, your body will replace the normal B cells, within six to nine months. Often, the disease comes back so we presume that the bad cells come back or may be left behind, and the treatment needs to be repeated. So, while your body is replacing those B cells you're more prone to infection and catching bugs – because the drug you used to kill the bad guys also killed the good guys,' Dr Leandro says.

'The data from the German group on CAR T-cell therapy was really amazing,' says Dr Leandro. 'The reports from their trial show that the patients experienced medium term remission: they responded very well, and they responded quickly. And much faster than what you'd normally see.'

The diseases that are being targeted now are ones where researchers know that B-cell depletion works, but that doesn't mean CAR T won't work well for other diseases.

'I suspect, that it will work very well in rheumatoid arthritis,' Dr Leandro says.

But why is CAR T working so much better than other drugs? One possible answer is that the rituximab was just preventing new plasma cells from forming, but it wasn't killing the existing ones quite as effectively.

'These trials may have taken the patient back in time, so to speak, to when they didn't have disease,' Dr Leandro says. That's huge. Taking your body back in time to BEFORE IT WAS SICK. But let's be clear: it doesn't mean that all the damage that's been done to your body by your disease will vanish, it just means that your immune system will be like everyone else's – that is, it'll stop making you sick, and just hunt down and kill bugs like the flu.'

There is, obviously, a huge amount of interest in these trials to see if they can reproduce the results from the original German study. There is also work underway in other countries, including China, and by the pharmaceutical company Novartis.

The other big question is whether it's worth it – physically and, sadly, financially. Are the risks of this kind of fast and severe depletion of B cells worth the disease remission they bring about? 'This is a treatment that is complicated, is costly,' Dr Leandro says.

The preparation and delivery of CAR T products is complex: you need experts from rheumatology, oncology and clinical trial delivery, to complete the process over several weeks.

The therapy used in this trial, called AUTO1/obe-cel, was developed at UCL by a team led by Professor Martin Pule

(UCL Cancer Institute) for the treatment of blood cancers like leukaemia.

'In the patients in the German group, the B cells came back at around three months,' Dr Leandro says. 'So we know that the CAR T cells are either exhausted or have completely disappeared. But it's a potentially life-long drug, isn't it? It's different from taking a tablet or giving patients an antibody that we know your body will clear eventually.'

And that's because the CAR T therapy can stay in your body for months and even years. Some may remain in the body as memory T cells, which can help fight the disease if it comes back. These memory T cells are what we count on with vaccines – they're kind of like the cells in our bodies that hold a grudge.

But to make the cells used in this treatment is time-consuming and expensive – it takes between 21 and 24 days to make the treatment researchers used in the UCLH trial. So this isn't exactly an off-the-shelf medicine yet.

And the procedure you have to undergo before you have the CAR T-cell treatment isn't exactly a picnic: to make space for the new cells, you have to take chemotherapy to clear enough space for these new T cells to expand and proliferate.

Then there are the side effects of the treatment itself, which can include cytokine release storms (when your immune system produces too many inflammatory signals, or to put it another way, starts freaking out – it can be anywhere from mild to severe). These can also cause fever, confusion, fatigue and nausea. Another potential side effect is something called immune effector cell-associated neurotoxicity syndrome (ICANS), which damages the brain or peripheral nervous system and can be caused by the engineered cells. It can happen right after cytokine release storms or several weeks later, and includes symptoms such as confusion, trouble staying awake or walking, shaking, and seizure.

But would it be worth it?

If you were in a bad way, and the CAR T-cell treatment would give you five years of remission, then, as Dr Leandro says, 'Certainly, for the more severe cases of lupus, particularly with severe renal involvement, which we know has a significant risk of morbidity and mortality, it may be a very good option.'

But beyond providing a potential new treatment, what this does is prove the concept that if you kill cells effectively, you can induce remission in lupus patients. 'You're essentially bringing their bodies back to the time before they developed disease. And if you have a remission period that lasts for five years, that's a huge thing,' Dr Leandro says.

Dr Leandro's team have done a lot of work on how to kill B cells better themselves. 'Instead of a live T cell that you might give to a patient, you're giving them an antibody that binds to something on the B cells. So it goes to the patient's system and uses the patient's own T cells to kill the B cells,' she says.

Essentially, it tricks your immune system into killing B cells by making them look like something your immune system would naturally want dead. And it works a treat, too.

Sadly for me, though, killing B cells isn't going to get rid of my AS. Yet. B cells have received relatively little attention in how AS develops, in part because there aren't any obvious autoantibodies to blame for the disease, but there's a growing body of evidence that suggests B cells are involved. And depleting B cells using rituximab showed 'beneficial results in a subgroup of patients with AS'.[2]

When I ask her what she thinks about the potential to use CAR T to treat my disease she looks a bit like I've put her on the spot. 'It's a very different disease,' she says. 'There's primary arthritis, where the disease presents mainly with inflammation in the joints. This includes seropositive rheumatoid arthritis which responds to B cell depletion. Then there are other primary inflammatory forms of arthritis that are called the seronegative or the spondyloarthritis group. This includes AS, and there's also psoriatic arthritis, which has multiple forms. Then there's reactive arthritis. But spondylitis is a completely different disease from rheumatoid. And anti-TNF inhibitors work for both,' Dr Leandro says.

So because anti-TNF works for rheumatoid and AS, then why couldn't CAR T?

Unintentionally, Dr Leandro reminds me how much I have to be grateful for: 'Anti-TNF inhibitors were a game-changer for ankylosing spondylitis. Before them we had nothing to offer. I started practising rheumatology

---

[2] https://pmc.ncbi.nlm.nih.gov/articles/PMC8703482/#abstract1

in 1993. The anti-TNF inhibitor trials started in something like 1994. It's brilliant having these medications, because before we had nothing to offer.'

Which is true. The anti-TNF inhibitors – my infusion, or maybe your epi-pen home injector Remicade or Humira – completely changed the way arthritis was treated. And it gave people with AS a treatment where before there wasn't much on offer.

It's important to be grateful. And I am. But can't we be grateful and curious and hopeful at the same time? I think we can.

YOUR BRAIN IS IN PAIN 3

'Pain's been good to me.'

By way of introduction, it sure sets a tone, but Chris Eccleston, Professor of Pain Science at the University of Bath, is serious. I'm not sure anyone who suffers from chronic pain would agree, but he's made pain his life's work. He's not alone.

'I've watched the whole business of pain grow,' he says. 'When I joined the International Association for the Study of Pain, there were around 400 people involved, now there are 8,000 around the world.' Which, he adds, isn't a lot for the size of the problem. The International Association for the Study of Pain is active in 125 countries, with 96 chapters and 25 special interest groups, and it's been going for over 50 years.

'There's one way of talking about this field, which is that it's very successful,' Professor Eccleston says. 'We do all the things you're supposed to do in the university and we're pretty damn successful. However, there's more pain than there's ever been before, and there are more people suffering from it, without anywhere to go and suffering in more and more complex ways.'

But why are there so many more people in pain now? People are living longer, for one. Which brings with it any number of complications, such as long-term health conditions that result in chronic pain. And there are significant changes to our lifestyles that bring chronic illness, which often brings along chronic pain: people who live with obesity and coronary heart disease, and complications from diabetic neuropathy, for instance. Then, of course, you've also got people who are living with chronic pain after successful cancer treatment, which is possibly the largest and growing group of people living with neuropathic pain.

The good news is that people are surviving cancer; the bad news is the treatment hurts. But we're all going to experience pain and how we come to that isn't what interests Professor Eccleston. What he's studying is how pain impacts on people's lives.

Which makes sense. If you're living with chronic pain, what does it matter how you got it? There's an acceptance that comes with living with chronic pain.

Twenty per cent of the population, adults and children alike, have chronic pain, but only one in five of those people have high impact chronic pain, leaving them with multiple disabilities or extensively disabled and distressed by their pain. But it's not clear why this is. How are some people able to find a way to live life in the context of pain and for others it is literally their undoing? What Eccleston and his colleagues at the Bath Pain Centre are doing is investigating this question; they are working to shift the field away from its relentless focus on intensity and the reporting of the sensation, and moving towards getting people to think about the impact of pain and how that affects the ability to live a good life.

To me, this mimics the process of adjusting to a new diagnosis of life with a chronic illness. There are steps you go through that mimic the steps of grieving. The majority of chronic pain researchers may be investigating the causes on the basis that if you find out what's causing the problem you can modify it so that it stops causing the problem, but knowing how you got your particular chronic pain injection system doesn't matter. You've got it and you need to learn to live with it.

But it's not as if Professor Eccleston doesn't want to see new pain killers being discovered; it's that while we're looking for one, and while we're withdrawing more and more analgesics from the market because they're harmful to people, or worse ineffective, then we need to do something else.

'The treatment goal should be to move people from high impact pain to low impact pain – to reduce the burden. We try to help people learn how to live with the constant threat of what can feel like catastrophic, unmanageable and inevitable consequences,' Professor Eccleston says.

His research group at the University of Bath has just had a paper accepted for publication in the flagship journal *PAIN* that looks at some ways of shifting that conversation. In it, they present a framework to be used to study states of chronic pain and the transitions between those states. Pain is dynamic in nature: it changes, ebbs and flows. The other thing this paper points out is the importance of incorporating the impact that pain has on a person's life. This is less about measuring the pain as it's experienced, and more about what pain does to your life.

For me, as a patient, the idea that pain isn't just something that affects your physical being, but your entire life – and those who are closest to you – feels almost revolutionary, because if we're only talking about how much it hurts on a scale of one to ten and where it hurts, then obviously we're going to focus on reducing that number. It's about correctly identifying the problem, and if you live with chronic pain, often that problem isn't just 'I hurt'; it's 'I hurt and life is difficult in these ways and impossible in these other ways'.

Why does it matter how we measure pain? It matters because we treat what we measure. You measure the problem, because whatever the problem is, that's what your doctors will try to treat. But pain isn't just a place where you hurt; pain's impact can be so much wider than that. For Eccleston it's about a different perspective: 'Whether a single brief event or a constant feature of life, pain interrupts to prioritise protection, interferes with activity, reduces quality of life, and can alter identity. Protection is achieved by escape from harm, avoidance of perceived danger, withdrawal for respite and repair, and communication of incapacity and environmental risk; longer term protection is achieved by learning the cues for pain and injury. From this perspective, pain is most usefully considered a need state, fundamentally a motivational drive to protect. This approach centres our attention on the consequences of pain for the person in their context, on its duration and its impact.'[1]

But being able to define the transitions between pain states – from acute to chronic – enables researchers to do a couple of other things, too. They can look at big data sets to look at the factors that range from genetic to psychological that can help predict the transition or lack of transition. The lack of transition is quite interesting because some people get stuck in a state of chronic pain. But why? This stickiness – which is what researchers call it when people are stuck in a place, with a lack of transition – keeps people in a pattern of behaviour that makes their life worse. If we can figure out what the cause is of people getting stuck, then we can predict when it might happen for other people, and if you can predict it then you can develop ways of preventing it.

There's a saying that goes, if it fires, it wires. Which means, broadly, that if you keep doing something, the pathway your neurons take to make that happen becomes entrenched. The same way a cut-across in a park becomes a path. People walking across it wear it down over time. The same thing – again, broadly speaking – happens in our brains.

But doesn't that mean the stickiness is permanent?

Not necessarily. Professor Eccleston tells me that we can rewire our own brains so that our chronic pain isn't a problem: 'One of the problems is that researchers have tried to

---

[1] https://researchportal.bath.ac.uk/en/publications/the-establishment-maintenance-and-adaptation-of-high-and-low-impa

apply an abnormal psychology, a science of psychopathology to pain, and it doesn't work, it doesn't fit because the way in which people behave when they're in pain is not abnormal. It is the opposite – it's hyper normal, in fact. People do all the things they have always done when they've had pain: they withdraw, they avoid, they ask for help, they take medications. The problem is that when the pain doesn't go away, we keep doing these things, even though they no longer help, and can cause further problems.'

The way to learn how to live with chronic pain is that you almost have to become countercultural. You have to start thinking about the world in a different way. Pain is a warning signal, a sign that you're in danger, but with chronic pain that's not the case, and part of learning how to live with it is learning how to ignore those pain signals.

This reminds me of what my old rheumatologist in Toronto, Dr Edward Keystone, told me. He said that my spine and hips were like the rusty hinges on a door, and if I didn't move them, they'd get stuck forever. He told me he'd give me whatever medication I needed to dull the pain enough to get moving again. Get back in the pool, is what he told me, essentially. You're in charge, you do the hard work, it's up to you. Not the kind of advice you really want to hear when you're in horrible pain and you're in your early twenties and feeling quite sorry for yourself. What I wanted was to hear that there was a tablet I could take that would solve my problems. I was prepared to be told I'd have to do stretches, which I knew I'd never do. I wanted to count on Big Pharma to save the day. How was I going to cure myself? I wasn't a doctor; I was a child who hurt. I'd spent my life swimming, and where had that got me? It seemed ridiculous to expect that swimming was now all of a sudden going to cure me.

The most annoying thing about all this is that it works. Professor Eccleston nods his head and says, 'Pain can become a signal to move rather than a signal to withdraw, but that takes a lot of hard work to learn to do that, to create these new relationships between signal and action. Some people learn to do this themselves, but we know very little about those people as we rarely meet them. But for most people it takes a lot of work.'

But the thing is that none of this has anything to do with the pathology – the study and understanding of how illness and diseases work and their impact on people. This is about the psychology (the study of cognition, behaviour and experiences, which differs according to social norms and rests upon a number of constructs that are deemed to be the social norm at any particular era). 'This is due to millions and millions of years of evolution that have driven this signal to alarm you and people around you to withdraw,' Professor Eccleston says.

He goes on to say, 'I think the other aspect of this is if we can focus on impact, then it might actually give us new targets for therapies, even new druggable targets.'

Usually, with analgesics or pain killers, you're told to stop what you're doing and think about your pain. Assign it a number on a scale of one to ten. Then a doctor will administer the analgesic and ask you to assign a number to your pain again, so if it's shifted from, say, a seven to a five, then you're good to go. A painkiller that reduces your pain is a good one, right?

But what doctors don't often ask is how does it impact your life? Because you have a life outside of your pain – or, at least, you did. According to Professor Eccleston, a good analgesic is one that, 'Doesn't distract you, one that allows you to get on with the world. We test analgesics by asking people to focus on the pain and rate it, give it a number. But a good analgesic is one that stops the pain interrupting you. One of the things we do is look at the effect the pain has on cognition, on attention, on memory and problem solving and reasoning. And a good analgesic is one that repairs your cognition and stops you from making poor decisions or improves your memory.'

Wait, my cognition is impaired when I'm in pain? I'm making poor decisions?

Professor Eccleston explains it like this: 'You're talking to me, but somebody behind you is tapping you on the shoulder saying, "Listen to me. Listen to me." Now you've got two things in your environment. You've got me talking to you, who is frankly really interesting. And then you've got somebody behind you who wants your attention and you've got to flip between the two things. You're doing very well at ignoring it because this is a really interesting conversation, but that person behind you really wants your attention, so they start hurting you. That's what it's like being in pain. And then suddenly you go, ohh, I missed that. What was that? And so you're not laying down memories because you can't pay attention. Your working memory is reduced.

Your executive function is reduced. In other words, your ability to really bring resource and stay concentrated on something is diminished. And all of those things then have real world effects, such as chronic pain patients make poorer financial decisions.

'It costs you money to be in chronic pain. So when you go to the shops and you look for the two for one offer and it says buy two, get one free or get two for one, or get 10 per cent off. It's quite hard to work those things out when it is hard to concentrate, hold information in memory, and switch between information.'

It's almost as if Professor Eccleston's been shopping with me. But what he's saying makes sense. When I think of what I'm like at work when I've got to push through the pain, I'm fortunate in that I can rearrange what I'm working on if I need to. Do something easy while I can't focus on much. Because the example he gives, of someone tapping your shoulder and then switching to hitting you, that's a pretty accurate description.

Professor Eccleston was the first researcher I met who's researching the role our brains play in our experience of pain, but he is far from the only one. The next researcher we're going to meet is looking at how our pain goes chronic – and how our brains are involved in that.

When did I first get a hint that I was in for a lifetime of pain? I don't remember it, but we had this cassette tape recording of my grandfather. In the background, you can hear me as a baby wailing. My grandfather helpfully pipes up – and you can tell he's joking – 'Oh, it's her arthritis! Her arthritis!'

Prescient or what?

I remember twinges when I was a child. One afternoon when I had been playing in our neighbourhood, I had to stop walking home and stretch out what felt like a tight muscle in my bottom and down the back of my leg. I don't remember much about the moment – it was just that, a moment – but I remember the location of the pain. My sitting bones. It was a weird place to hurt. It's not like I'd been skating and fallen on my bum or anything. It was summer. I stretched it out a bit and carried on. I don't think I mentioned it to my mom at all. But now, with the benefit of hindsight and a diagnosis, I wonder if that was the start of my arthritis.

But what if the circumstances of my childhood made me more likely to go on to develop chronic pain? I mean, I have a disease, which I didn't get from having a hard childhood. But with chronic pain, as I'm learning, there seems to be a lot of different knobs you can fiddle with. I'm imagining it sort of like a sound board – but it might be easier to imagine it more like an outfit. You can dress it up or dress it down in a lot of different ways, and everything makes a contribution – some bigger than others.

I had, by most measures, a pretty good childhood. We lived in a nice house, in a nice neighbourhood – I had friends, my siblings and I got on really well, we had fun pets. We had holidays and grandparents and trips to the movies. We had swimming and figure skating and soccer. Art camp and piano lessons. Homemade cookies.

The only black mark was my parents' divorce, which was ugly and messy and involved a lot of shouting. Before they even got to the divorce stage, there was evening after evening of arguing and horribleness. My father euphemistically referred to these evenings as discussions with my mother. Suffice to say that news of a divorce wasn't the letdown they were expecting. Did that have an impact on my pain, or how I process it?

I don't know. But what I've learned is that adverse childhood experiences (ACEs) may affect how the brain processes information, including pain. Young people with lower brain efficiencies that were exposed to more ACEs have pain symptoms comparable to youths with chronic pain.

What are lower brain efficiencies? It means a decreased ability in places like your brainstem and cerebellum to process information really well. Your cerebellum is in charge of motor movement regulation and balance control; it also contributes to cognitive processes and even emotional regulation. What that means is that those brains need to work harder to do basic functions compared to a normally functioning brain. That might lead to slower responses, impaired coordination, or difficulties with automatic bodily processes – the stuff your body does without you having to think, Hey, go and do this now.

Understanding this relationship between ACEs and pain is important because it might help us to identify pain symptoms earlier, particularly in vulnerable populations such as young people who've been exposed to trauma. The really important thing is that it's critical for preventing the chronification of pain.[2]

---

[2] https://onlinelibrary.wiley.com/doi/full/10.1002/ejp.4702

You read that right: preventing it from going chronic.

Dr Melanie Noel is Professor of Clinical Psychology at the University of Calgary in Canada. She reminds me instantly of a woman who was one of my extra moms when I was growing up – the kind of person you could call when you got into trouble and who would come and get you, no judgement whatsoever. The kind of person who doesn't mind being woken up in the middle of the night if you need help – someone who sees their own ability to help as a gift, not one for you or me, but for themselves. We speak first thing in the morning, her time, and she's just coming back from a serious injury, but she's full of energy, and enthusiasm, and excitement. She is an absolute joy to talk to. What's more, I get the feeling – right away – that she's exactly the kind of researcher we want on our side.

She's a psychologist and she primarily works in paediatric pain. Her research interests include questions like, 'Why pain becomes a problem, and why it transmits through generations over time? Why do the things that happen to our parents and our grandparents – whether that's trauma, adversity or pain – get under our skin and influence the next generation? Why does that happen? How?'

To understand all that, we need to look at societies and cultures. How do our social worlds, media, culture and systems of oppression drive pain and what are the possible antidotes to that? 'I focus on children, but I really look at lifetimes and generations upon generations and in terms of development,' Professor Noel says.

Studies suggest that about one in four or five children and adolescents experience headaches, abdominal pain and musculoskeletal pain, and the rates of paediatric pain are actually rising. Beyond being a rising public health disaster, researchers know that once chronic pain develops, especially at critical developmental periods in childhood and adolescence, it can really rob children of a typical development, and influence their cognitive, social and emotional development. And, of course, this has a massive impact on families.

But the interesting thing to Professor Noel is what happens when those children grow up. Researchers know that of young people who have chronic pain, up to two-thirds of them will become adults with chronic pain if they don't get the right intervention when they need it. But even if those children get treated well and doctors get rid of their pain, those children are at an increased risk for developing things like anxiety, depression and PTSD when they become adults. Her research group has also shown that chronic pain in your teenage years increases the risk of developing opioid misuse problems into adulthood.

Professor Noel became interested in more pathological forms of memory, like PTSD, and when she looked at the literature, it had been known for decades that there were alarmingly high occurrences of PTSD symptoms and chronic pain in adults. But these things had never before been examined in young people. She and her research team compared a group of young people who had chronic pain and a group who didn't, and their parents, and asked them about PTSD symptoms. Almost a third of the children with chronic pain had clinically elevated levels of PTSD. Her research team also found that 16 per cent of the parents with children who had chronic pain had clinically elevated PTSD. Compare this with a recent study from King's College London that shows that one in thirteen children have had PTSD.[3]

But why? When we think about PTSD and chronic pain, there's an idea that there should be a traumatic injury that leads to chronic pain. The pain is a reminder of the trauma. But when Professor Noel and her team asked people about their traumas, they talked about things like the death of someone they knew, physical illness or hospitalisation, as well as emotional abuse.

They looked at all the literature to try to figure out what the factors are of these shared vulnerabilities, as Professor Noel calls them, might be that lead to the development and maintenance of both these problems. They made a model where they looked at factors in the children, and from both PTSD and chronic pain, there seemed to be shared risk factors: avoidance, memory biases, depression, hyper arousal and sleep disturbances. Those last two things were coming through in the literature as being really important to the exacerbation of both problems.

Then, working with colleagues in neuroscience, they looked for potential genetic and epigenetic (how our behaviours and environment can cause changes in the way our genes work) reasons for the development of PTSD and chronic pain. They knew that of parents of children with chronic pain,

[3] https://www.kcl.ac.uk/news/troubling-extent-of-trauma-and-ptsd-in-young-people#:~:text=New research from King's College, irritability, impulsivity or difficulty concentrating.

about half of them had chronic pain themselves and a lot of them also reported experiencing trauma.

They also followed children over time. When children came into the clinic with higher levels of pain that was getting worse they had higher levels of PTSD and their pain and disability got worse over time. And this points to the importances of those PTSD symptoms in making pain worse over time. Keep in mind that PTSD symptoms are symptoms of trauma.

Next, the researchers looked at adverse childhood experiences (ACEs). These can include physical, emotional, sexual abuse, neglect, household dysfunction, and they can also include someone in the household that had a mental illness, a relative in jail, a mother being treated violently, substance-abuse problems in the household, and also separation and divorce. Another researcher, Dr Vincent J. Felitti, Clinical Professor of Medicine at the University of California, had already shown that the higher level of ACEs you had, the more likely you were to experience alcoholism, drug abuse, suicide attempts, depression and, more shocking, you were more likely to have life-threatening physical health problems like heart disease, cancer, chronic lung disease, skeletal fractures and liver disease. This showed then that these ACEs really set the stage for mental and physical health problems down the line.

Professor Noel's group wanted to see what the prevalence of ACEs were and what the influences of ACEs were in their paediatric chronic pain patients. About a quarter of their patients reported that someone in the household had a mental illness, one in four were saying that they had parents who were separated or divorced; there were also relatively high levels of emotional abuse and physical violence in the household. But then they wanted to know if this increased level of ACEs for the children also indicates an increased risk for poor outcomes, and, not surprisingly, it does.

They found that children who have higher levels of ACEs, particularly three or more, report lower quality life over time. They report greater symptoms of major depressive disorder, they show higher levels of PTSD.

But what she shares next is really encouraging. Professor Noel tells me about a paper ('Positive childhood experiences and chronic pain among children and adolescents in the United States'[4]) that looked at positive childhood experiences and resilience, which are things that act as buffers to the negative effects of trauma. There are seven things that researchers include as positive childhood experiences: the ability to talk to your family about your feelings, feeling that the family was supportive in difficult times, enjoying taking part in community traditions, feeling a sense of belonging in high school, feeling supported by your friends. You had at least two non-parent adults who cared about you. And you felt safe and protected by an adult at home. Essentially, did you have social support and people who were there for you when you were a child?

---

[4] https://pmc.ncbi.nlm.nih.gov/articles/PMC10330007/

The study looked at adults with high levels of ACEs and those were linked to worse mental health and socio-economic outcomes over time. The higher level of positive childhood experiences people had were buffers against the ACEs. They were the antidotes.

So this is really mind-blowing: to prevent chronic pain in children from turning into chronic pain and worse in adults we need to give those children more social support. They need people to count on, people who are going to show up for them. And right there, we can stop that pain from becoming chronic.

Does that sound unbelievable to you? It sounds crazy to me. I ask Professor Noel if this is possible for people like me, who have a musculoskeletal disease.

'You can talk to someone about their pain and that can change their whole life,' she says. 'Being validated, being believed, being connected, having community – that is not fluff. That can actually change the trajectory of someone's life.'

When Professor Noel mentioned being believed, I told her a bit about how I went from being in a lot of pain, to having a name for that pain. I was living in Toronto at the time, and my GP was my grandmother's old GP, Dr Hussein. She was possibly the best GP I've ever had – she always listened, deeply. She oozed empathy. My sister and I would both happily wait an extra two or three (sometimes four) hours in the waiting room to see Dr Hussein. We waited because we knew that everyone got as much time as they needed while Dr Hussein listened to your problems.

I told her how my bum hurt, my sitting bones, how I walked with a cane. I burst into tears on her a few times, especially when I was telling her how I just couldn't sleep. She assured me – she looked me in the eye, she smiled, she probably hugged me and rubbed my back – that we would get to the bottom of this. That she wouldn't stop until we knew what the problem was. And she didn't.

I've been pretty lucky with doctors, and I can't imagine what it must be like for people who haven't been believed. When Dr Hussein told me that she wasn't going to stop until we figured it out, I believed her. I knew she would do everything – and more – to take care of me.

She sent me to a couple of rheumatologists and none of them were a great fit, but Dr Hussein kept referring me until I found one I clicked with. He was a rheumatologist at Mount Sinai in Toronto, called Dr Ed Keystone. This guy changed my life.

Or, as Professor Noel tells me, 'He's the hero of your story.' He told me he couldn't cure me, per se, but he could make me feel a hell of a lot better. He'd give me whatever pills I needed to ease the pain enough to get back in the water and start swimming again. I did as he said, and it worked. I started swimming again, and got rid of my cane.

Professor Noel asked me why I believed Dr Keystone. I have to say, I'd never really thought about it. The question flummoxed me, to be honest, so I listed off a few things I loved about him, and Professor Noel smiled knowingly. I just knew, I told her. I just knew he cared about me.

'How did you know?'

'He made eye contact,' I said. 'He asked me about myself. I felt like a person, not a chart of diseases.'

Professor Noel nodded vigorously. 'He gave you validation. He brought humanity, and he validated you. That is what validation is. It is conveying to the person that you care, that you understand, that you see them. He is the hero in your story.'

She goes on to add, 'And how could he have shown you that, had you not told him your story? You couldn't just walk in and expect to feel that connection. People like that, they change lives. When you can root the turning point in your story to one doctor, who listened, who put his pen down, looked at you and said – not just the words because it has to be authentic – but who says, "I believe you." That's everything.'

She's absolutely right. It is everything. She tells me that it's all about story and relating, being present and doing exactly what Dr Keystone did for me: he listened to my story and gave me empathy.

This idea of being listened to as a patient comes up a lot when I talk to my fellow chronics – and something one of them said really stood out to me. I asked if people had anything they wanted the medical community to know. One respondent, SM, said she wanted the medical community to listen: 'To actually listen to what people are saying and don't just write them off because they don't have a medical background. Don't assume we don't know what we're talking about because we're not medical doctors. I really do feel that if people had listened to me from the start, it wouldn't have taken me as long as it took to get a diagnosis. I feel that not being believed and not being listened to … I think there's a real trauma in not being in control of your own body, and then also not being believed about your own body.'

This idea that pain is connected to so many other aspects of our lives is at the heart of what Professor Noel is doing to dissect the culture of pain. I ask her to clarify whether she means physical or emotional pain, and her answer comes at me fast and is so good that I want to share it in its entirety.

> 'You cannot have debilitating physical pain without having a wild emotional experience, and vice versa. You can't have PTSD or depression and anxiety and not have physical pain. Things are so connected! Processing trauma can bring forth physical pain and psychological pain. Living a life with pain can, in and of itself, be a trauma, right? And why is that? Because for some reason in our society empathy fails for some people, but why, when and for whom?

But we were talking about preventing that transition from acute to chronic pain. Where does empathy come into that?

Forty years ago, the problem was that for babies requiring surgery (more often than not preterm babies) there was a question of balancing removing that pain through anaesthesia and the very high inherent risk of anaesthesia for those newborns because monitoring vital signs was rudimentary and the issue with foetal blood meant that anaesthesia had a very narrow therapeutic window between consciousness and death. What really wasn't known so much then were the long-term consequences of that early life painful intervention. Now, we know that those experiences are felt and remembered – not always in detailed, verbal accounts – but crucially, they can actually change brain development. They can set the stage for pain all the way through into adulthood.

By validating a child's pain, you might be able to reduce their distress and consequently their pain, so they have a more positive experience around pain and injury. It also helps to teach them how they can regulate their emotions appropriately in these kinds of situations.

Validating can help prevent bad memories of pain – and it's those bad memories that can lead to pain problems and avoiding healthcare in the future. Validating a child's pain can really help them to understand their emotional and physical experiences around pain and injury, and when that doesn't happen, it can lead to them mistrusting their own pain experiences.

When a child feels they're believed about their pain, that builds trust. They know they can talk about their painful experiences and that they'll be believed and supported. This is of course a good thing, and I'd imagine what every parent would want and hope to do for their child. The really interesting thing is how much of an impact that can have on your child's future. This is an 'untapped, modifiable social pathway that could have significant implications for the understanding, treatment, and prevention of chronic pain in the next generation'.[5] It seems like something so easy to implement that we'd be foolish not to – and as a

[5] https://journals.lww.com/pain/pages/articleviewer.aspx?year=2024&issue=12000&article=00004&type=Fulltext

non-pharmaceutical intervention probably comes with fewer potential side effects too.

Professor Noel says, 'How do you move people's hearts? How do we not get desensitised to other people's suffering? And you've seen it with doctors, everyone living with pain has experienced this. And I believe the only way we can change this is by changing different parts of our culture. And we can do that through stories.'

She continues, 'Everything is story. Story is medicine. Stories bring us together. And stories of other people who have had these illnesses or these conditions matter. Those stories can liberate, but they can also tie us down. And stories are always changing. Yes, pain is pain. We focus on the suffering, but if I can relate to you through my story and that can evoke empathy and validation, then I have community in you, and that's my path to healing.

'How we talk to each other about pain and our journey and our story, that can set us free. Some of my closest friends live in debilitating pain, and at some point they were burdened by it, but not now. So, understanding how we tell these stories can completely transform our experience of pain.'

But it's not just the stories we tell; it's the culture in which we live that matters, too. 'I'm obsessed with culture because we can look at parents and children, and we can look at clinicians and patients, but we're all human beings affected by the culture. It's the patriarchy, white supremacy and capitalism – none of these help us in being communal and showing up for each other and believing each other,' she says.

Professor Noel was, when we spoke, recovering from a bad accident that necessitated surgery. She praised the opioids that doctors gave her saying that they saved her. Then she corrects herself: 'Do you know what actually saved me? It wasn't the opioids. No, it was my dad flying down to help me with my kids. My neighbour cooking me food. My best friend sitting in A&E to advocate for me.'

It's community care too, and how do we foster communities that can support that? 'Pain should be the great unifier,' she says, like a rallying cry. 'We socialise empathy out of society, and then we ask why is society like this? We've got a cultural problem.'

She goes on to tell me about a way of thinking that's focused around narrative, called, appropriately, narrative medicine.

Here's my confession: part of me is really dubious. But Columbia University in New York has a division of Narrative Medicine. Here's what the handbook says: 'Narrative medicine is a fresh discipline of healthcare that helps patients and health professionals to tell and listen to the complex and unique stories of illness. Arising at Columbia University in 2000 from roots in the humanities and patient-centered care, narrative medicine draws patients, doctors, nurses, therapists, and health activists together to reimagine a healthcare based on trust and trustworthiness, humility, and mutual recognition.'

'The goal of narrative medicine from its start has been to improve healthcare,' says Rita Charon, an internist and literary scholar who is the founder and director of the Program in

Narrative Medicine at Columbia University, in which future doctors and medical clinicians are taught how to elicit, interpret and act upon the stories of their patients.

Is narrative medicine going to make my back stop hurting? Probably not, but it might help your doctor to have a little more empathy for you and that might actually make you feel better – emotionally at least, which might have physical implications.

I spoke with Olga Torres in New York who teaches the subject at Columbia. 'The way that I found narrative medicine was that I live with six autoimmune diseases, including a rare disease, scleroderma,' she says. 'I have lupus. My type of lupus means that I have no control, I can't open anything. I can't hold a fork. The nerves stopped wrapping around my muscles.'

She teaches virtually, typing is excruciatingly painful, and she's on three kinds of biologic medicine. Her lupus is at the stage where she's eligible for the CAR T-cell therapy that started me on this journey. She has two friends who are doing the CAR T-cell therapy and both are doing really well.

After Ms Torres survived and recovered from a brain injury (which took six years), she returned to law – her previous occupation was as a public defender – and she realised she needed to do something else because her life had changed completely: 'By the time I could win a case for my clients, they were too sick to take advantage of the treatment, or had died, which was quite depressing. And then a friend told me about narrative medicine.'

Narrative medicine uses the principles of attention, listening and reciprocity to help medical providers better hear patients' stories of illness. 'Not symptoms,' she emphasises. '*Stories* of illness.' What she means is that she wants doctors to not just listen for what's coming out of a patient's mouth, but to see the patient, notice what they're doing with their body, so that hopefully they can understand a bit more about what that patient might be leaving out of their story. The idea is that it helps doctors acknowledge biases and prejudices.

Because maybe when the doctor encounters someone who is, for example, asking for pain medication, they think, 'I've had too many of this type of patient come through the emergency room,' and they treat them according to that bias, not according to the illness or unique patient. The hope is that, with practice, clinicians can become better at spotting those blindspots for themselves, and that will help them to see patients as more than a collection of symptoms.

'It's about simple things like doctors not standing over patients, instead sitting down and looking them in the eye. It's about taking the time to say, "I'm sorry about this horrible experience you've had,"' she says. When writing down someone's story, doctors are encouraged to share what they've written with the patient and to ask if they've got that person's story right.

There are three key points to all this: attention, representation and affiliation. They want doctors to actively listen, to co-create the medical history with the patient, and hopefully with enough trust, patient and doctor create a bond and have a productive relationship.

Now, it seems to me that this is all pretty obvious, basic stuff. But there's a moment when some doctors – not all – put on the white coat and begin to think that they're superhuman. The point of it is to get doctors to be better listeners and encourage them to work together with patients when making decisions – especially about long-term illnesses. It's also for patients, to help them to tell their own stories so they get better or more appropriate care.

This all really chimes with Professor Noel's research around the stories we tell ourselves about our pain, and how those stories have a direct influence on how we cope with our pain.

'The field of pain has been dominated by Western, male-led theories,' says Professor Noel. 'That permeates how we think about and conceptualise it. When a patient has a complaint, doctors try to understand that to find the cause. The "cause" that we have the evidence to see. And then we find the thing that fixes the thing and so on. But pain doesn't work like that. It's highly individualistic,' she says. 'Why do we believe that someone's sad or scared, but we don't believe that someone is in pain? It should be the one thing that we can all identify with in some way. It should be the great unifier. We all experience it,' Professor Noel says. But instead, it's socialised out of us.

Another societal amplifier of chronic pain is isolation, which is quite worrying when you look at these statistics: In 2022, 49.63 per cent of adults (around 26 million people) in the UK reported feeling lonely occasionally, sometimes, often or always. And around 7.1 per cent of people in Great Britain (almost 4 million) experience chronic loneliness, meaning they feel lonely 'often or always'.[6] In Great Britain, between one-third and one-half of the adult population, or roughly 28 million people, is affected by chronic pain.[7]

But the thing that protects – even in the face of things like abuse and neglect and adversity – is community, the opposite of isolation. This means having people in your life that show up for you, people that can take you to the doctor, who love and validate you, that you can talk to about difficult things, that you enjoy community traditions with. And that's great for lots of obvious reasons, and also for a slightly less obvious one. My partner so often wants to 'do something to help', but beyond bringing me my heating pad and a few tablets, there isn't much he can do. Being part of my community and doing all those things we listed off above, that actually does really help. And that's kind of amazing.

Professor Noel isn't the only academic who wants to understand how our early life experience can – or cannot – set us up for a lifetime of pain. Her collaborator, Professor Richelle Mychasiuk, Department of Neuroscience, University of Sydney, Australia, focuses on how early experiences modify brain development in adolescence.

Professor Mychasiuk started off by looking at parental stress and early life enrichment, and drug exposure, trying

---

[6] https://www.campaigntoendloneliness.org/facts-and-statistics/

[7] https://cks.nice.org.uk/topics/chronic-pain/background-information/prevalence/

to learn what might make people more susceptible to learning disorders or mental health conditions. But then she met Professor Noel, who suggested she look at pain, and she's now looking at how early life experiences contribute to susceptibility to chronic pain. She wants to know what happens in the brain when an acute painful trigger transitions to chronic pain. Because most people get better, they don't go on to develop chronic pain. So what makes us so special?

And what about people, like me, who have a genetic disease as the reason for our pain? And what about people who've had an injury that's healed but still experience pain? 'Early life trauma primes the body to be hyper-reponsive later in life,' Professor Mychasiuk tells me. 'Regardless of whether the injury has healed, or whether there is ongoing inflammation or the disease is ongoing, the early life adversity basically changes the starting point – your baseline health. If you think of it as a scale, and you have to tip the scale with so many things to develop chronic pain, early life trauma is one of the things we add to the scale. Then your injury, other life factors, genetics all also pile onto the scale. Positive things, like good pain management, social support, good mental health, they all go on the other side of the scale.'

She's researching the role cytokines play in pain. Cytokines help control inflammation and they allow your immune system to mount a defence if germs or other substances that can make you sick enter your body. Too many cytokines can lead to excess inflammation and autoimmune diseases. So, Professor Mychasiuk asks questions like, if a mother experiences trauma and her oxytocin levels change, does that change the baby's circulating levels of cortisol?

Oxytocin's a hormone that plays a role in reproduction, social behaviour, and stress and anxiety. Cortisol is your body's natural alarm system. It's the primary hormone involved in stress response and works alongside certain brain regions to regulate your mood, motivation and fear.

It suppresses inflammation, maintains blood pressure, raises blood sugar levels, regulates your sleep-wake cycle and boosts energy to manage stress, helping to restore equilibrium once the stress has passed. During times of stress, it also shuts off systems – like your digestion – to focus energy where it's needed. Cortisol provides anti-inflammatory assistance too, as part of the preparation for any tissue repairs needed. Your brain tells your adrenal glands when to make more or when it's time to stop making cortisol.

'Prenatal stress primes your immune system to be hyper-responsive or hyper-reactive. So normally, if you didn't have that experience, a typical inflammatory response if you had your tonsils out or scraped your knee, your body would deal with that and move on. But if you have a hypersensitive immune system from this early life trauma, your immune system overreacts. It's kind of like an allergy, an over response because of that initial stress or injury and it takes longer to go away,' she says. This all creates a learning mechanism where now your brain is pairing those two things together.

But not everyone who has chronic pain would have experienced this kind of early childhood/prenatal trauma. Professor Mychasiuk's research group has also studied trauma using the model of intimate partner violence, which looks at combat-induced trauma in dads who are military veterans, and the PTSD they deal with. There are other models that look at the things that have the biggest effect, for example putting rats on a high-fat, high-sugar diet, which completely primes your immune system to be in a hyper-inflamed state that sets your offspring up to be more susceptible.

I guess that good nutrition could be classified under resiliency factors. And what Professor Mychasiuk has found is that there are enough resiliency factors to offset a lot of these adverse early childhood experiences, especially in today's society where we have access to education and nutrition advice. Not all people will have access to everything, of course. Talking about excessive caloric intake, she says, 'It's a balancing act, right? You're eventually going to tip the scale one way or the other, but I don't think that we're helping – I think we're setting children up to have to overcome hurdles for no reason.'

Resiliency is good, but what would be even better is not having to be resilient in the first place, so if we can learn how something goes from acute to chronic, we can then figure out how to stop that process. From the research that Professor Mychasiuk and her group are doing, the idea is that when you take away the context of injury, then what's actually driving the pain is more of a psychological effect.

'It's basically a learning mechanism,' she says. Your brain has put stress together with being in pain, so lucky you, now every time you activate your stress response, your body signals pain. In the same way you learn a bad habit, or develop an addiction, your brain has learned to pair these two things together, and the more often it pairs them, the more often the neurons fire together and you end up with a stronger and stronger connection between these two things.

How do you fix it?

'To fix it, you have to unlearn it, and unlearning something is harder than learning it in the first place,' she says. For example, if it took three years to get to that point where your pain has become chronic and your brain's circuits have been rewired, then it's going to take at least three years to unwire those connections.

So how do we actually invest the time or get people to invest the energy to unlearn those connections or those improper relationships? 'I think when we have these situations like trauma or these high fat diets that prime the body, prime the brain to be more susceptible, it makes that learning and that pairing stronger, and it makes it happen faster. I think that it all contributes, but the best way to explain it is improper learning, because that's what your brain is doing. Everyone thinks learning is beneficial, but it's not always good.'

We have a fear response for a reason, so we don't put ourselves in danger. We don't do stuff to ourselves that will cause further damage. But at some point, when, for example, the inflammation's gone and the body's done all it can and it's stopped sending those pain signals – what if you've paired walking upstairs and your back hurting? Then every time you see a stairwell, your brain goes, 'Hey, don't do that. Remember what happened last time? It hurt.'

'So then you've generated this fear now that you've associated stress and pain, and it just triggers the same,' Professor Mychasiuk says. 'Your body really has only a few ways to tell you not to do something. For instance, if you think about eating something awful: you're gonna throw up – because that's the mechanism your body has to get rid of stuff. So you get that nauseous feeling for so many things because that's how your brain says, Don't do that. Your brain is like: I know if I make you feel nauseous, you won't do that anymore. There's only so many ways your brain can tell you to stop, and pain is one of them.'

Just because your brain is telling you that you're in pain, but there's no injury, does NOT mean it's psychosomatic or that you're making it up. 'It's 100 per cent there,' Professor Mychasiuk says. 'We know from imaging studies that we've changed wiring in the brain, you've changed neural circuits in there, but it's not because you're actually in pain, if that makes sense.' It means that we've trained our brains to be in pain. So even though the inflammation is gone, or the injury has healed, our brains are still shouting PAIN. And if your brain is in pain, then so are you.

Can we unlearn those connections? And even if we can, I mean, who has the time and energy? Is that really what you want to do when you're in agony?

A colleague of Professor Mychasiuk's is using virtual reality (VR) to help people do this exact thing. Say you have something that's normally painful to do, for example going up the stairs. You put the VR goggles on and, in the VR world, you re-learn how to go up the stairs. She starts you off with little stairs and they eventually get bigger. For people with complex regional pain syndrome where anything hurts – like touching their hand makes it feel like fire – in the VR world, they'll put their hand in different things and it doesn't elicit that pain response. So they can start to teach their brain that not everything is painful. This way, people are getting that continuous feedback that this doesn't actually hurt. The scenarios are changing for them and their brains are too.

Professor Mychasiuk suggests that if we added something called transmagnetic stimulation (TMS) to this VR work-out then we could really be on to a winner. They're already doing case studies and trials on it in chronic pain – it's also been used to treat depression. TMS uses magnetic fields to stimulate nerve cells in the brain to improve symptoms of major depression. It's called a 'noninvasive' procedure because it's done without using surgery or cutting the skin.

'TMS increases plasticity in the brain. I think if you could pair this TMS with something like virtual reality, you could speed up the unlearning process, so it wouldn't take three years to unlearn these patterns involved in chronic pain,' Professor Mychasiuk says. Basically, this is a way to say to your brain: It is OK if you do this, you won't be in pain. And then your brain slowly learns that, and it stops triggering that pain response. The more you do it, the more you build the neural pathways, and your brain learns, just like it learned the other way.

'I don't think that it's going to bring us to a point where you'll be pain free all the time. But I think that it would definitely help a lot of situations where you have an over-response stress response to things. That's the part that we could really provide benefit for,' Professor Mychasiuk says.

She's spent the past five years developing models to induce chronic pain, which are to understand how it works, and now she wants to fix it. Her research group does a lot of work with epigenetics and changes in gene expression. These are changes that – unlike genetic changes – are reversible. They change how our bodies read a DNA sequence. And Professor Mychasiuk has identified several new diets that could change methylation patterns and impact how genes are turned on and off. Methylation is the chemical modifications of DNA that happen when methyl groups are added to DNA. The patterns can change during development and cell differentiation.

Now, I'm no stranger to special diets. As a child, I had one. My siblings and I struggled with various things – reading, concentration, maths – and our mom tried everything with the doctor, specialists and all the rest, until she wound up at the door of an allergist. From there were spent a lot of years on a variety of weird diets, which generally had in common the exclusion of wheat, dairy, sugar and corn. I grew up in Canada, where to avoid those foods is no mean feat. But those diets helped. When we didn't have any sugar or wheat or dairy in our food, we were able to sit still and concentrate in class. This was a pretty big win.

Along with these restrictive yet effective diets, my siblings and I were signed up to competitive swimming and figure skating and soccer. The idea was that we'd be able to focus if we just burned off some of that energy. I mention this all because when I hear what Professor Mychasiuk is saying about being on high-fat, high-sugar diets priming your immune system to be hyper-inflamed, it's no wonder our allergy diets helped.

But what Professor Mychasiuk is also saying is that they know when you have exposure to these early life stressful events that you get methylation of genes. The genes are essentially turned off or other genes get turned on and they're working in overdrive. Other researchers have been looking at diet supplements with things like folic acid, vitamins B6 and B12, and other ways to try and change gene expression for the better.

At the moment, this work is happening at a genome-wide level – which means whatever researchers do affects all the genes. They need to do a lot of RNA segmentation work to understand which genes are being turned on, and to uncover if those are involved in pain or anxiety and so on. Once they have a better understanding of those then they can target them specifically.

'I think it's also going to be age dependent because you don't want them to always be on or always be off. We'd need to regulate that along with maturation. We know that to develop mentally, you need stress, but just a bit of stress.

Same with the genes. We need them to be Goldilocks – as in, just right,' she says.

Here's another example of why early life matters. Professor Mychasiuk was interviewed for a documentary about a man who was sexually abused as a child. He went on to develop chronic pain and couldn't get rid of it. He saw something like a hundred doctors, and none of them were really able to help him get rid of that pain. So he started doing that thing that all of us with chronic pain have done: he started doing his own research and realised that his trauma was probably contributing to his pain. He did the work to deal with the psychological trauma and the pain went away.

'I think something like that is just such a remarkable story – it wasn't all in his head,' says Professor Mychasiuk. 'It was definitely driven by his brain. But his brain was putting up these warning signals for a reason that had nothing to do with what he thought it had to do with. I think that your brain does a lot more than we give it credit for. And I think that it's super protective for evolutionary reasons even if the way it does that doesn't always make sense to us. I'm not saying that always dealing with trauma will fix everything. But I do think it doesn't hurt.'

Researchers used to think that people with mental health issues developed pain problems, but what they're finding now is that – in children – it's actually pain that's often what's leading things like opioid misuse. Pain in children is leading to anxiety, to depression, insomnia. And even suicide.

'Pain can kill,' Professor Noel says. Her research group published a paper[8] last year showing that eleven-year-olds who had a parent with a mental health issue 'are at risk if they had pain. Only nine months later, they were more likely to develop suicidality.' That's as astonishing as it is disturbing. And it makes me thinks that we're not taking pain anywhere near as seriously as we need to be.

There's another huge predictor of future pain: maternal separation. It's one of the worst traumas you can experience, and researchers use it in animals to model early life trauma. Any serious and prolonged disruption of parental care, especially in infants and very young children, alters how the young brain develops. Children under the age of five who are separated from their parents find that they can't depend on their presence and care anymore, and that causes their stress levels to spike. As stress hormones rise, they change the physiological functions of our bodies to help us cope with threat. But these prolonged increases in the levels of stress hormones disrupt physiological functions and cause inflammation and epigenetic changes – chemical alterations that disrupt the activity of our genes. Turning genes on or off at the wrong time changes brain development and, importantly, it changes how our neural networks are formed and how different parts of the brain communicate with each other.

Studies show that the separation from parents causes a rapid maturation of brain circuits responsible for processing

---

[8] https://pubmed.ncbi.nlm.nih.gov/38719156/#:~:text=Abstract,b = 6.96, P =.

stress and threat. This changes the brain's wiring as well as the way emotions are processed. These studies also show that it doesn't take long for separation to hurt.

In lab studies of animal models, we know that the stress caused to the rats is because of the mother's absence – for the rat pups that's the only thing that changes.

Brain imaging shows the structural and functional changes in the brains of children separated from their parents. We can see that the amygdala (which is used to process threat and emotion) increases in size, and its connections with other areas of the brain are altered.

This separation also changes the expression of receptors on the brain cell's surface that are involved in stress response and emotion regulation, which disrupts communication between neurons.[9]

Terrifying? Yes. But Professor Noel suggests that they're a clear way forward to combat this (beyond the obvious that we should never separate children from their parents, unless they're at risk): 'We're even finding in the animal and the human you can wipe those negative changes out through community, through social support. If those children get that social support. This is why we really need to think of the society and the culture of pain, too.'

If you think about certain cultures, Indigenous people in Canada who were brutally separated from their parents and sent to residential schools and thereby forcibly separated from

---

9 https://theconversation.com/a-sudden-and-lasting-separation-from-a-parent-can-permanently-alter-brain-development-98542

their parents, or people trying to emigrate to certainly the United States or other places, we're creating a generational pain issue. What happened where you live, what the colour of your skin is, what happened to your mother, your grandparents, your ancestors – that all plays a role in your future, and your future experience of pain.

'But to me,' Professor Noel says, 'it's pretty freaking amazing that we are finding that – even in the face of being locked and loaded with all of that – that there's actually a way to turn it around for the next generation. And that's what gets me really excited. The question is how do we shift the culture? This should be an area that everyone can see themselves in. More than any other, because everyone is going to have pain, everyone.'

I want to know how we can get these ideas into policy. Imagine if we could stop a lot of chronic pain before it starts? And in the case of miserable diseases like mine, or fibromyalgia, then surely living in a culture that has more empathy, where doctors are better at listening, and where we use our stories to tell ourselves how great we're doing – I think that should be such an easy thing to do. I think that if there is a magic bullet, maybe it's this, these ideas around culture and understanding the root of chronic pain.

But for chronic pain to take hold, there has to be an insult or stressor of some kind. Dr Simon Beggs, Associate Professor, Developmental Neurosciences Department at UCL's Great Ormond Street Institute of Child Health, is looking at a lot of the same things that Professor Noel is, but from a different perspective. The Institute of Child Health is a kind of link between UCL and Great Ormond Street Children's Hospital: at the hospital, he leads on preclinical research in the paediatric pain research group. What this means is that he can take the conventional research route – taking cutting-edge research from the lab and trying to use it in the clinic – but also the reverse, taking clinical observations and modelling them in the lab to try to get an insight into the underlying cellular and molecular mechanisms, something that can't be done in human patients. He's looking at how our earliest life experiences influence our experience of pain, and in particular chronic pain.

He works closely with Dr Suellen Walker, Professor of Paediatric Anaesthesia and Pain Medicine at UCL's Great Ormond Street Institute of Child Health, who has pioneered the study of pain in neonates (a newborn up to the age of 28 days) and what lasting effects that has on chronic pain in adulthood. These are the premature babies who, because they're born so early, are unfortunately exposed to all sorts of painful things as part of their neonatal intensive care. Things like even having their heel poked to take blood every few hours and high rates of surgery, because just by being born early, we know there's something wrong, and what they're finding is that it's actually the act of tissue damage that's setting these children up to be primed for a lifetime of pain. 'She was the first to really identify this group of really vulnerable infants who were born very early, who undergo surgery, and how this impacts their outcomes in later life,' Professor Beggs says.

The thing about newborns is that their developing nervous system is more susceptible to changes in neural activity, so pain in early life may produce effects in newborns that it wouldn't in older children. As a result, early tissue injury may lead to 'persistent changes in somatosensory processing and altered sensitivity to future noxious stimuli'. Which means that all this pricking – which is necessary to help these newborns – might actually lead to changes in how they process sensation, and it might change their sensitivity to painful stuff. There's growing evidence that newborn pain can result in long-term changes in emotional and rational behaviour.

'From our animal studies, we showed if you have a painful event in early life that influences your pain in later life. To the extent that a very small injury like cutting your hand, which to us as adults, would be a few days of mild discomfort and then it's fine, actually has a much greater degree of discomfort of pain, and it lasts much longer simply because it was something done to you as a newborn,' Professor Beggs says.

Just a tiny little incision under anaesthesia in a hind paw in the mouse, and that will lead to a bit of extra sensitivity for a few hours. And then by the next day, they're fine and you can barely see the scar. And it's a very minor thing. But Professor Beggs and his team showed the same thing happening when the mice grow up. 'So in this case, it's two or three months later, and there's no sign of any incision. They look completely normal. But if you perform surgery again, their response to a painful event in adulthood is much more exaggerated,' he says.

Researchers have done these kinds of models with things like stress, too. One of the explanations they came up with for the exaggerated reaction in adulthood was because the painful stimulus occurred at a time when both the nervous system and the immune system were still developing. That primed the immune system to react in this hypersensitive way – it's not designed to experience pain like this. The immune system responds inappropriately because it's primed – almost as if it learned from that first experience – so it has a bigger response. That's the theory behind things like juvenile arthritis – adolescent disorders that appear around puberty because it's a stressful time.

But once you make it out of puberty, then what?

'One of the big aspects of chronic pain in adulthood is that it's not simply a sensory event experience. Researchers can show you have a heightened pain response, but if you talk to patients with chronic pain, a lot of them talk about things like their sleep disturbances, anxiety, depression, a lack of motivation, and social withdrawal. And a lot of patients say that the sensory aspects of pain are not necessarily top of the list of things they struggle with. If you could make me sleep better, that would go a long way to helping. All of those things are part of it. The sensory aspects of pain don't exist in isolation,' says Professor Beggs.

I always refer to the things outside of the pain itself as 'cope factor'. If you've got enough cope factor, you can deal with the pain. Lack of sleep and fatigue are the things that make me feel like I can't cope with my pain if I'm in a bad flare, and, of course, pain is something that causes you to have a terrible sleep, so you feel fatigued, and so on into the vicious and miserable cycle.

'If you look at the definition of pain that the International Association of the Study of Pain uses, it's a sensory and emotional experience. Not every painful event has an emotional aspect to it – it's not just a sensation, it's an experience. I'm particularly interested in the experience of it. So if your early life experience changes your sensory response to pain, does it also affect things like anxiety, sociability?' Professor Beggs says.

This may mean that, if my immune system is primed for a fight, my emotional responses are too. 'If the primary immune system is causing an increased pain response, then your increased pain response is going to be associated with bigger emotional aspects as well,' he says. I wonder if it makes us have heightened emotions – and then, if we go back to Professor Noel's ideas around empathy, does that make us maybe slightly more empathetic? I'm not sure it's the kind of thing a researcher would want or need to investigate, but I do wonder.

These painful early life events change the structure of the brain. Researchers have documented these changes using MRI and they've found changes in parts of the brain – the amygdala – that are associated with things like fear and anxiety. As part of Professor Walker's EPICure UK cohort,[10] researchers looked at nineteen-year-olds who'd had surgery as preterm babies, and they found that the volume of amygdala is different. Professor Beggs says, 'It would be a big leap from saying this means that part of the brain now functions differently, but it's clearly been affected – it's smaller or shrunken. This

[10] https://www.bjanaesthesia.org/article/S0007-0912(18)30336-2/fulltext

was particularly the case in the girls rather than the boys. And the girls showed higher anxiety and the boys didn't. So there's a correlation between anxiety behaviour, sex difference, and the volume of the amygdala.'

That is wild. Why does the reaction appear more pronounced in girls over boys?

'That would suggest that the immune system is not necessarily directly involved. But there is the fact that the early life experience has changed the brain, and the subsequent development of the amygdala. Which we showed in the mouse models,' Professor Beggs says. 'And we can go back to when the mice are just ten days old and predict their anxiety behaviour in adulthood just from that, because the changes are already there.'

His results are preliminary. They don't know why this is or what it is exactly that's behind it because they're just doing MRI, which only shows that there's a volume change. 'Is that volume change the number of neurons, number of immune cells, the vasculature?' Professor Beggs asks. 'We don't know. It's a big question, but the volume is definitely different and the volume is associated with behaviour in later life. It seems like with the emotional aspects of this, that the changes that are required are set in place very early. So what we're trying to do is figure out if there's something we can do to prevent it.'

One of the ways they're doing that is to look at the microglia, which is the central nervous system's immune system. They knew that for pain, in a developing immune system, it had something to do with the actions of the microglia. If the preterm baby undergoes a surgical incision, then when they grow up and have a subsequent surgical incision, their pain responses are amplified. Professor Beggs showed that if you block the microglia (drugs can create a temporary block) at the same time as the adult incision, you can block that pain response.

But then they did it the other way around, blocking those cells at the time when the rodents were preterm babies. Researchers gave the tiny newborn rodents a blocking drug while they underwent surgery. The pups grew up and when they received a repeat incision, the pain effects were completely blocked. The primary effect is gone – but only in the boys, not the girls.

He gives me a minute to pick my jaw up off the ground, and then rewinds back to the 1990s and tells me about the typical way researchers would do a mouse experiment in a neuroscience lab. They'd choose a young adult male mouse as their model. 'You only had to use a few of them and you'd get nice results because they all behaved the same.'

A lot of researchers missed the sex difference because they weren't actually testing females at all. It's only in the last ten years or so that we've seen a big push to reflect society in experiments which are made up of men and women. 'You need to have both male and female mice, and still people are not doing it,' Professor Beggs says.

I presume researchers don't want to include female subjects because of our hormone systems. 'But it's not necessarily anything to do with it. That's just a lazy assumption,' he says.

What his research group are finding is that the more they look at this stuff, the bigger the sex differences are. 'Which is good because we know that there are these big sex differences in the clinical population. Things like IBS and Crohn's are very, very heavily weighted towards the female population,' he says.

In the USA, the National Institutes of Health (NIH) created a task force about this because there's been a big problem with translating pain research – and that problem is the translation just isn't working. 'I gave a talk to the medical students yesterday, a lecture about pain, and there was a big meta-analysis of pharmacotherapy for persistent post-surgical pain,' Professor Beggs says. 'Persistent post-surgical pain is a big clinical problem. People really don't realise that there's a fairly hefty minority of patients who undergo surgery, routine surgery, open heart surgery, hernia repair, all these different things, who end up suffering from chronic pain. Pain that may still persist two years afterwards and be untreatable. It's a big problem. And, of course, every year there's millions of these surgeries happening. So the problem is only getting bigger.'

The Cochrane Group is a global, independent, non-profit network of health researchers and professionals, patients and carers, and in 2013 they did a survey of chronic pain. It was a meta-analysis of all the drug treatments for the prevention of chronic pain after surgery in adults. The report looked at all the evidence for things like gabapentin, pregabalin, non-steroidal anti-inflammatories, intravenous steroids, all NMDA blockers, intravenous fentanyl, intravenous cytokine, inhaled nitrous oxide – and none of them work.

'If you look at them rigorously, none of them work. And their conclusion in 2013 was, and I quote here, "additional evidence from well-designed large scale trials is needed in order to more rigorously evaluate pharmacological interventions for the prevention of chronic pain after surgery". That was 2013,' Professor Beggs tells me.

Duly noted. They did the survey again in 2021.

'And again, they say despite agreement that chronic post-surgical pain is an important topic, extremely little progress has been made since 2013, likely due to study designs being insufficient to address the complexities of this multifactorial problem. And they conclude with, "based on currently available evidence, none of the drugs studied so far can be recommended for clinical use specifically for the indication of preventing chronic pain post-surgery".'

Professor Beggs lets me sit in stunned silence for a second.

'Let me understand this,' I say. 'We realise there was a problem. We didn't deal with it. It remains a problem. We can't treat it.'

Professor Beggs says, 'Yeah.'

There's a big problem in the translation of pre-clinical science to clinical interventions. Essentially in turning research results into new drugs. 'You can get all these amazing results in a laboratory setting, but as soon as you try and create a drug, and go through drug trials, they fail,' Professor Beggs says.

Take for example immune inhibitors for pain (a drug like Remicade, for example). The research was done in male mice and it worked beautifully. Then researchers took the drug to clinical trials and they gave it to a random sample of the population, which is half men and half women. Because they hadn't done the pre-clinical work on female mice, it didn't work.

Another reason why it's so hard to develop new drugs is the placebo effect, especially in pain research. Professor Jeffrey Mogil, E. P. Taylor Chair in Pain Studies at McGill University in Montreal, did a review of the clinical trials. So, in a clinical trial, if you want your new drug to be approved, along with showing that it's safe, obviously, you have to show that it has an effect greater than placebo. 'That's the first hurdle – if you don't get higher than placebo, it's a non-starter, and it's been noted that, particularly in pain research, the placebo effect has been getting bigger since the 1970s or so,' Professor Beggs says. Professor Mogil looked at all the trials in the world (around pain drugs) and at the placebo effect. And he found that the increase in the placebo effect is driven by trials done in America – and that's the key part, America. This change in placebo treatments for pain holds true only for US clinical trials.

'We were absolutely floored when we found out,' said Professor Mogil. Simply being in a US trial and receiving a sham treatment now seems to relieve pain almost as effectively as many promising new drugs. He thinks that as US trials get longer, larger and more expensive, they may be enhancing participants' expectations of their effectiveness. 'Based on patients' ratings of their pain, the effect of trialled drugs in relieving symptoms stayed the same over the 23-year period – but placebo responses rose. In 1996, patients in clinical trials reported that drugs relieved their pain by 27 per cent more than a placebo did. But by 2013, that gap had slipped to just 9 per cent. The phenomenon is driven by 35 US trials; among trials in Europe, Asia and elsewhere, there was no significant change in placebo responses.'[11]

Professor Beggs tells me that part of the reason for this is that there's so much money in the US – because at the moment, the treatment options are opioids or anti-inflammatories. 'There's no other drug treatment. Those have been used for ages. The quest for a new painkiller is massive; in terms of a market leader, this is going to be billions of dollars, and the drug companies are putting everything they've got into these trials.'

He paints a vivid picture: If you were to participate in a trial, you'd be met by a very shiny person with very white teeth and a nice crisp lab coat with a glossy brochure about their new drug that's going to cure your pain. And you'd believe it. Then the placebo effect goes through the roof, and that's specifically in American trials, where this is how the trials are run, as opposed to over here, in the UK, where it will be some overworked lackey in a lab coat saying, 'Next!'

Professor Noel also pointed out the placebo effect to me, as something that – to her way of thinking – really highlighted the power of story to achieve results: 'The power of language, the power of social context – the placebo effect is one of the greatest achievements of modern medicine in some ways. But it's almost magic, that for some types of pain, some types of headache, for example, they've done trials and shown

---

[11] https://www.nature.com/articles/nature.2015.18511#:~:text=A basic principle of these, risen by the same amount.

that placebo is as or more effective than the greatest drug we have, amitriptyline.'

I've taken amitriptyline and I'm not sure I'd say it's the greatest drug we have, but it did knock me out and I cared substantially less about my hideous rib pain. But the placebo effect is more than positive thinking. It's creating a stronger connection between the brain and body, and how they work together.

Check this out: 'Placebos won't lower your cholesterol or shrink a tumour. Instead, placebos work on symptoms modulated by the brain, like the perception of pain. Placebos may make you feel better, but they will not cure you. They have been shown to be most effective for conditions like pain management, stress-related insomnia, and cancer treatment side effects like fatigue and nausea.' That's from Harvard Medical School.[12] And those are some of the conditions that we chronics suffer with.

Researchers still don't totally understand how placebos work, but it involves a complex neurobiological reaction that includes increases in endorphins and dopamine, and more activity in certain brain regions linked to moods, emotional reactions and self-awareness. A study published in *Science Translational Medicine* tested how people reacted to migraine pain medication and placebos. One group got a migraine drug with a label giving the drug's name, the other group had a placebo with the label that said placebo. A third

---

[12] https://www.health.harvard.edu/newsletter_article/the-power-of-the-placebo-effect

group got nothing. Researchers found that the placebo was 50 per cent as effective as the real drug in reducing pain after a migraine.

For a placebo to work, you also need the ritual of treatment. You go to a clinic at certain times and you're examined by medical professionals in white coats. You receive all kinds of exotic pills and undergo strange procedures. All this can have a profound impact on how the body perceives symptoms because you feel you are getting attention and care.

Getting attention and care are the important things to point out there. That's empathy, isn't it? And it's exactly what Professor Noel was talking about.

But we need new drugs. Professor Beggs told me about a new one called Journavx that just passed its FDA approvals, but only for acute pain. It's a sodium channel blocker, which works in a similar way to lidocaine but is specific to the sensory part of the nervous system. If you were to block all sodium channels, you block motor functioning as well, which you don't want.

The drug company that makes it, Vertex, says that the drug 'blocks pain signals only found in the periphery, not in the brain', and that it's not addictive. It's been approved in the USA for the treatment of adults with moderate-to-severe *acute* pain. The company is also evaluating the drug to treat peripheral neuropathic pain, diabetic peripheral neuropathy and sciatica.[13]

---

[13] https://news.vrtx.com/news-releases/news-release-details/vertex-announces-fda-approval-journavxtm-suzetrigine-first-class

But back to our immune systems. In 2018, the NIH put together a task force of the great and the good of pain research in America. And they asked, 'What's wrong? What do we have to do to treat all these people in pain?' That delivered two recommendations: we have to be more aware of early life experiences because, in pre-clinical lab studies, researchers are looking at an experimental animal as an adult, in isolation, and assuming that's the same as a human patient in isolation, which is not the case. 'Your pain biography is going to influence your pain responses,' Professor Beggs says.

Secondly, you have to look at women as well as men. 'I mean that seems like a stupid thing now, but they had to actually reiterate that. And NIH then went and changed their policy. And if you have funding from NIH, you have to include female subjects in your experiments,' Professor Beggs says. (We spoke before President Trump's policy that instructed the NIH to not approve grants that include words such as 'women', 'trans' or 'diversity'.[14])

It seems reasonable to think, then, that your early life experience influences your pain, or maybe your predisposition to chronic pain and also other parts of your pain experience – for example, comorbidities associated with your pain. And there are differences between men and women which are due to fundamental differences in how the immune and nervous systems interact.

---

[14] https://www.pbs.org/newshour/health/what-happens-to-health-research-when-women-and-diversity-are-banned-words

But the thing that Professor Beggs thinks is 'probably the biggest thing that's going to happen' is mining the wealth of information we have and using it to define experiments. 'But again, if you're a patient with chronic pain, no one asks you about what your pain experience has been. You're not going to be asked by your doctor, Were you born early? Did you have surgery as a child? It's not on a medical record. We don't know the pain biography of a lot of pain patients and that's not taken into consideration at all,' Professor Beggs says.

If we're heading towards more personalised medicine, which seems to be the case in specialities like cancer, then we need to have a lot of this background information. 'How do I know that you've got an immune system primed for pain, that you've had this earlier surgery that's going to influence how a drug will work or what your responses to pain are? We know that if you have open heart surgery for a bypass – a standard bypass which millions of people in this country will do every year – 30 per cent of them will suffer from intractable, persistent post-surgical pain two years later,' he says. So what is it about the other 70 per cent – what do they have that the others don't? 'I would suggest that at least part of that is due to early life experience.'

Others might argue otherwise, but if these early childhood experiences are going to have some influence, then wouldn't it make sense to include them?

'Only by understanding these early experiences, and then if we can, mapping the changes that occur using mouse models as I've been doing, can we see when the changes start,' Professor Beggs says. 'My preliminary results suggest we may be able to predict anxiety behaviours associated with post-surgical pain as early as ten days old (in mice). The best way to combat this is prevention at the time of the initial surgery, but again, if that's an immune component, it's tricky thing, because you don't really want to be targeting the immune system as a treatment. In that case, maybe targeting specific parts that are responsible for that is the way forward.'

And it makes so much sense, doesn't it? But then, if we know this stuff, why aren't we doing it? Knowing that these things are underway is a step forward. It means that, as an adult, the reason you're responding differently to surgery is because your brain has been changed by your early life experiences.

Some of those differences are because your immune and central nervous systems have been changed because of what's happened to you in your life – in the same way that your socio-economic environment will also change you. Do you live in a place of high pollution? Do you have a very stressful life? Is your diet not particularly great? The epidemiology is very complex, but outside of that researchers can isolate what it is about this early life pain experience or pain exposure that is clearly having an influence.

That's a complicated big picture. 'The psychologists will tell you it's all about psychosocial factors. And the neuroscientists will say it's something else. And that's a big thing to try and get a view of. Professor Noel will say that you've learned pain differently,' Professor Beggs says.

I suggest that maybe he's focused on internal things, and Professor Noel is more interested in external influences.

'They all need to be taken into consideration. And there's more than one way of looking at it, so it's about trying to draw things together. Recognising the importance of both and how one influences the other. It's a weird idea that psychology is outside of biology. It's quite strange to silo it by asking, is it a biological effect or psychological effect? What's the difference? Yeah, it's a psychological effect, but it's still nerve cells and molecules that are underlying all this. It's a biological process, but the outcome is different.'

Another researcher who is interested in pain and the brain at perhaps its most fundamental level is Dr Prasad Shirvalkar, Associate Professor of Anesthesia at the University of California, San Francisco. He's a neurologist and 'a pain and systems neuroscientist' he tells me when we speak first thing in the morning, the day after the 2024 American presidential election. 'I see patients for pain management, where I perform nerve blocks and neuromodulation – spinal stimulators and that sort of thing,' says Professor Shirvalkar. 'In the lab, my work is running clinical trials to try to understand if we can develop a new therapy using brain stimulation either invasively or non-invasively. We don't understand pain processing in the brain as well as we do other fundamental things like vision. Pain is much more complex than a primary sense, but we don't even understand that as well as mood or depression.'

His lab is running a clinical trial that involves the invasive surgical implant of wires in people's brains to find out what region works best for them as far as pain reduction goes. They'll use this information to detect biomarkers of each person's individual pain states and pain fluctuations, and then implement them in a kind of personalised algorithm to stimulate unique parts of the brain at personalised time points to really to try to help patients.

In parallel, they're trying to develop a non-invasive treatment with focused ultrasound, which is obviously much less invasive and risky. How does it work? 'Ultrasound has always been an imaging tool where we can put a transducer on any body part to try and see through the shadows by using acoustic signals,' he says. 'Newer systems have used high-intensity ultrasound, which can emit multiple sound waves at different frequencies and different angles that can interfere with one another. The idea is with high-intensity if you use a thousand different elements – you can have the sound waves interfere and actually heat up tissue and destroy it or ablate it. That's high intensity but with low intensity you can do a similar kind of thing without heating up tissue and modulate electrical activity in the brain. We don't yet know the parameters or which sound frequencies and intensities do what to the brain's electrical activity. We're still figuring out the basics – but this is happening in humans, using prototype devices. So in the future someone could put on a helmet with a computer programme and we might be able to shut down a part of the brain.'

Right now, Professor Shirvalkar and his lab are planning to use high-intensity ultrasound in specific brain areas for specific disorders. For pain, they're starting a clinical trial to try to find good targets and identify the right phenotypes for the syndromes they would have the most success treating.

The hard part is, unlike using a more invasive technology, researchers can't get a direct read out of brain activity in real time.

Professor Shirvalkar has a strong interest in fundamental neuroscience and the computational processes in the brain. 'My lab is hoping we'll get funding to study brain behaviour quantification,' he says. 'How do we quantify the brain's behaviour? We have all these signals – like heart rate, for example – and we can capture more signals than we are capturing right now. But can we quantify just through people's behaviour or physiological or behavioural states when someone is in a high pain state? Can we develop predictive biomarkers just based on behaviour and then try to understand: how does the brain at a network level undergo those switches in states?' The answer is not just yet, but Professor Shirvalkar and his lab are working on it.

'I want to understand what the basic features or structures are – these networks that exist in the brain – and then figure out how they switch. What are the dynamics? And then relating the two, how does the brain change at the network level? How does that relate to behavioural changes and what are the mechanisms there that are causing that to happen?'

If they can figure that out, then they might be able to determine what the differences are that lead to pain or reflect chronic pain, and then how researchers – and doctors – like him can actually help. 'By help I mean how can we influence or modulate these brain state changes to prevent and/or treat pain in folks who have it, to ideally prevent pain formation in the first place?' he adds.

As far as applied research goes, they're conducting a small clinical trial. 'We're starting to just understand what brain targets to stimulate, how often we need to stimulate them in order to treat neuropathic pain – things like lower back pain. We're trying to understand how we might develop treatments for syndromes that have poor or limited options,' Professor Shirvalkar says.

Another focus is understanding how technology that helps spinal cord stimulation and peripheral nerve stimulation for pain works. 'I want to know why they work, when they work,' he says.

The understanding of how and why and when things happen – this is part of what people mean when they talk about basic or fundamental discovery science. We need to understand these things to come up with new treatments or even cures. 'I was talking to David Julius who won the Nobel Prize in 2021,' he says. Professor Julius, Physiology Chair at the University of California, San Francisco, investigated how temperature is translated into nerve impulses. He used capsaicin, a compound from chili peppers that induces a burning sensation, and DNA fragments, genes, which are active in heat-sensing neurons. One single gene was able to make cells capsaicin sensitive. Further experiments revealed that the gene encoded a heat-sensing receptor on the neurons. 'He keeps emphasising the point that we really need to understand the basic mechanism, the fundamentals of what pain is,' Professor Shirvalkar continues. 'We don't even know how visceral pain from the colon gets transmitted to or interpreted by the brain. We have some idea of what nerves are involved with the autonomic nervous system, but we don't know much about the autonomic nervous system in comparison to the somatic nervous system. So he would say that we need a basic understanding of life, the biology and the anatomy. I think people working in in those fields often don't get recognised, especially if their work doesn't have a clinical application. I think that there's a lot of value in doing the basic foundational research.'

He's right. There is. It's the foundation of what we know about our bodies and our diseases. And it's that knowledge that serves as the building blocks for treatments and cures.

SEX DIFFERENCES IN PAIN 4

An article on the American Association of Medical Colleges website states: 'Throughout history, doctors have considered women's bodies atypical and men's bodies the "norm", despite women accounting for nearly half the global population and outnumbering men in the United States since 1946. Though policy and social changes in the 1990s have helped turn the tide, women remain underrepresented in research, sometimes grossly so.'[1]

When I spoke to some fellow chronics as part of my research for this book – the majority of whom were women – one of the questions I asked was what they'd like to see in terms of research from scientists. The overwhelming plea was for research to focus on women and our health. As one sufferer, AP, puts it to me: 'I remember telling two doctors that my symptoms always got worse around my menstrual

---

[1] https://www.aamc.org/news/why-we-know-so-little-about-women-s-health

cycle and they said, "No, it doesn't." And my pain flaring up was quite often how I knew my period was coming, but the doctors told me it wasn't that, but was something else. I just kind of felt that was a bit off.' She was being so much more polite than I'd have been if my doctors had told me that.

Another fellow chronic pain sufferer, KA, puts it to me like this: 'Throughout my life, I've gone to doctors and I point out a side effect or a symptom I've had, and the doctor disregards it and says whatever I've noticed or experienced isn't part of it. And I don't know if their research has always been inclusive enough. Has it always included women? Has it included women of all ages, because something seems to be missing from the bucket. For instance, I was 100 per cent sure when I tried the birth control pill in my twenties that I was having side effects from that, and then both my sisters had it. But all of our doctors didn't believe us. We stopped taking the pill, and our side effects went away. I feel like that still happens. I'm pretty in tune to my body. I know how I'm feeling and I know what's normal and what's not normal for me. And I'd like for researchers to start studying women's hormones. Maybe start there and then it's not so scary to have to factor that in. Maybe if we just understood it a bit better, that would also be less frustrating. Maybe if menopause wasn't this big question mark in everyone's minds, including the medical community, maybe we could have some concrete answers about it and not just live in this veiled haze of menopause, but we don't really know what that means.'

In 2024, the International Association for the Study of Pain focused on sex and gender differences in pain, to bring greater awareness to the area within the pain community and beyond. They stated: 'The 2024 Global Year will examine what is known about sex and gender differences in pain perception and modulation and address sex- and gender-related disparities in both the research and treatment of pain.'[2] In the same year, the Women and Equalities Committee presented a report that looked at women's reproductive health conditions, and while they didn't look at pain – chronic or acute – they did find that getting a diagnosis and treatment can take years, which leaves women and girls to endure pain and discomfort that interferes with literally every aspect of their lives. All those undiagnosed, untreated conditions also usually get worse while waiting around for someone to take them seriously.

Again, and even though this is focused on exclusively female conditions, it really rings true for chronic pain (which women experience more than men – 70 per cent of people who experience chronic pain are women[3]). 'Pervasive stigma associated with gynaecological and urogynaecological health, a lack of education and "medical misogyny" have contributed to poor awareness of these conditions,' the report concluded. 'This is mirrored,' it added, 'in a lack of medical research, treatment options, specialists, and the de-prioritisation of

---

2 https://www.iasp-pain.org/advocacy/global-year/sex-and-gender-disparities-in-pain/#:~:text=IASP is designating 2024 as,address sex as a variable

3 https://www.health.harvard.edu/blog/women-and-pain-disparities-in-experience-and-treatment-2017100912562

gynaecological care as evident by waiting lists, which have grown faster than any other specialty in recent years.'[4]

The report also cited 'the severe pain experienced by some women undergoing routine healthcare procedures such as hysteroscopy, IUD fitting and cervical screening'. It called on the NHS to do more to monitor and enforce protocols governing such procedures and ensure they are underpinned by informed consent, are trauma-informed, and take account of a patient's medical history and related experience. The NHS, it added, should collect data on whether guidelines for potentially painful gynaecological procedures are being adhered to, including patients' experiences.

Data collection is all well and good, but it doesn't directly address the issue that women's pain isn't being taken seriously enough, that woman aren't getting the pain relief that we need, when we need it.

I'm not the only one who thinks along those lines. A group of researchers collaborated on a paper that was published in *PAIN* (2021). The title of their paper was: 'Pain in Women: A Perspective Review on a Relevant Clinical Issue that Deserves Prioritization'.[5] That report noted a few really interesting areas where a lot more in-depth research is needed.

For example, testosterone deficiency has been linked to a high risk of inflammation in the nociceptive nervous system;

[4] https://committees.parliament.uk/committee/328/women-and-equalities-committee/news/204316/medical-misogyny-is-leaving-women-in-unnecessary-pain-and-undiagnosed-for-years/

[5] https://link.springer.com/article/10.1007/s40122-021-00244-1

diet and nutrition are factors that influence the perception of pain; the association in chronic pain with anxiety and depression puts a strong emphasis on common neurotransmitters – and therefore shared mechanisms – between these conditions in women.

Though there is a lot of data available, it's not stratified by sex. If it was, there would be an opportunity to better understand differences between the sexes in pain relief and beyond, including how other treatments work, which, in turn, would have an impact on pain. For example, treatments that target ankylosing spondylitis target specific molecular pathways, but research shows that some treatments, such as IL-17 blockers, appear to work better in men than women.[6]

The authors of the paper point out that: 'It is essential that different specialties collaborate to develop gender-related diagnostic and therapeutic guidelines.' They end the paper by saying that at the moment there are no drugs to manage chronic pain that have been specifically developed for women. And that, besides migraine where monoclonal antibodies have been developed, treating chronic pain is mostly managed using drugs that were developed for other diseases (for example, depression and epilepsy) that have limited effectiveness and aren't well-tolerated. The WHO's 'ladder for cancer pain relief', which lists paracetamol, NSAIDs and codeine as first and second rungs on the ladder, is still what doctors use today to guide treatment for chronic pain. 'New drugs

---

[6] https://spondylitis.org/spondylitis-plus/sex-differences-in-ankylosing-spondylitis/

are in the pipeline and will hopefully broaden the options in the future, but they are not yet available for use in the daily battlefield of our outpatient departments. Although a new approach to targeting treatment specifically by gender may be possible based on studies on the interaction between the immune system, inflammation, and pain, we are still very far from a pain treatment which is specifically targeted to gender-related pain conditions.'

That feels pretty discouraging. But I suppose, on the bright side, at least now, in 2025, we're looking at gender differences, so we're not starting at complete rock bottom. The sex differences researchers have found in pain biology, though they may only represent a 'fraction' of all those that exist, are nonetheless extensive. 'The biological processing of pain, regardless of how much pain is produced, is dramatically sex dependent. Different genes are being used in both sexes – different proteins, different cell types, dramatically different biology in each case,' says Professor Mogil. He did a review of the existing literature and found that at least 49 genes or proteins have been implicated in chronic pain processing for male (but not female) rodents. And 35 genes or proteins have been implicated in female pain processing but not in male rodents.

The reason for the longer male list? In part because of the biased history using male research animals. A report entitled 'Investing in the 51 percent' written by the NHS Confederation says that male bias extends to the very foundations of our health and social care system in the UK, which was 'designed around a white, cis-gender, heterosexual, male prototype'.[7] And the UK stands out as the country with the largest female health gap in the G20 group of nations, and the twelfth largest globally.[8] Here, women spend THREE more years in ill health and disability as compared to men. The 'male default' permeates research, clinical trials, education and training, as well as the design of policies and services. Gender bias in medicine is not only scientific or biomedical, but also social, cultural and political. And as Professor Watt, who we will soon meet, points out, there is an intersectionality of biases around chronic pain, female health issues, ageing processes, being older together with biases around common musculoskeletal conditions that can be dismissed as a normal part of ageing or in some way inevitable.

Evidence suggests that healthcare staff routinely underestimate patients' pain, and particularly women's pain, based on a number of biases and beliefs that have little to do with their actual testimony. A study in 2008 looked at the underuse of total joint replacement in appropriate candidates, which is more than three times greater among women than among men. Physicians, when asked, said that the patient's sex had no effect on decision making, however, the results of the study say otherwise: 'In total, 42% of physicians recommended total knee arthroplasty to the male but not the female standardized patient, and 8% of physicians recommended total knee arthroplasty to the female but not the male standardized patient. The odds of an orthopedic surgeon recommending

---

7 https://www.nhsconfed.org/publications/womens-health-economics

8 https://www.benenden.co.uk/gender-health-gap-2024/

total knee arthroplasty to a male patient was 22 times that for a female patient.'[9]

In 2016, Professor Amanda Williams at UCL conducted a study to look at whether clinicians' pain estimations were affected by patients' depression history and their 'trustworthiness' – an automatic judgement we make of other people's faces. Women's pain was underestimated by both men and women.

The gender bias holds true even when observers are watching the same expression of pain. In one simple experiment, observers watched a video of a five-year-old having blood drawn from a finger, expressing pain. Observers for whom the child was described as 'Samuel' rated the child's pain higher than those for whom the same child was described as 'Samantha'.[10]

'Given that women with chronic pain greatly outnumber men, to ignore female-specific pain biology is to do a great ethical disservice to the majority of people with this condition,'[11] writes Professor Mogil. An ethical disservice is the least of it. If women and our different bodies aren't taken into account when new treatments and drugs are being developed, forget the fact that you're going to lose a massive market, it's just not OK.

Remember when Professor Eccleston said that being in pain was expensive? The economic impact – in the US

---

[9] https://pubmed.ncbi.nlm.nih.gov/18332383/

[10] https://www.ucl.ac.uk/news/2021/apr/analysis-womens-pain-routinely-underestimated-and-gender-stereotypes-are-blame

[11] https://www.nature.com/articles/nrn3360#Sec2

alone – from some of the top players include: chronic low back pain, $100 billion; IBS, $380 billion; endometriosis, $22 billion; and fibromyalgia, $20 billion.[12] Though those numbers include men, they're also pain conditions where women are over-represented.

But this is about more than medical misogyny. There are actual biological differences in men and women, and that has huge implications for our experiences of pain. Even our immune systems are different. Immune cells play a key role in pain transmission and the development of chronic pain. But evidence is increasingly showing that these cells and pathways are different in males and females. In male rodents, pain depends on: microglia, purinergic receptors and brain-derived neurotrophic factor (BDNF) signalling. Or, to put that in a slightly more digestible way: a lot of brain stuff. And in female rodents? Chronic pain depends on the infiltrating T cells of the adaptive immune system.

Professor Mychasiuk's lab does a lot of work around sex differences, and they've done work where the behaviour of a male and female rat is the same, but then when researchers look at the inflammation profile and gene changes, the male and female rats are completely different. In female rats, neuropathic pain is associated with higher CGRP in the brain. CGRP (calcitonin gene-related peptide) is a protein that helps control blood pressure by expanding your blood vessels, but if you have migraines, your body makes extra CGRP, and the

[12] https://www.iasp-pain.org/resources/fact-sheets/gender-differences-in-chronic-pain-conditions/

excess activates nerves in the brain that make pain signals worse. Drugs acting on CGRP have recently been approved for the treatment of migraine, and analysis of the clinical trial data suggests that these drugs are only effective in women (the drugs in question being ubrogepant, rimegepant and zavegepant). 'So a drug that helps a male by increasing CGRP, for example, is going to do nothing for a female, but I think that's where we're actually going to make the biggest immediate impact. It's low hanging fruit,' Professor Mychasiuk says. Here's another crazy thing about CGRP – when it's applied to the surface of the rodent brain it produces pain hypersensitivity only in female mice.

A number of explanations for these sex differences in pain have been suggested, and they range from sociological to psychological and biological. Some show that sex differences are essentially an artefact. Take, for example, pain scales. If you've got chronic pain you'll be familiar with this: ten is blacking out, worst pain imaginable. But could this pain experience be affected by childbirth? Since men don't give birth, that pain doesn't come into their ideas around worst pain ever. So does that mean that for women, our pain scale, our ten, is bigger? And if that's the case then would that also mean that a woman's five is a more painful than a man's five?

Men are encouraged to be tough – to man up, to be a man, to suggest a few gendered expressions – and not to show pain, but for women it's OK, almost expected. This might lead to biased reporting in one sex and not the other.

Professor Mogil believes that 'the evidence for both clinical and experimental sex differences is overwhelming, it is true that the clinical impact of this research is very limited'.[13] He thinks this is because researchers are focused on studying quantitative sex differences in pain – meaning sex differences in the amount of pain (or analgesia) observed or reported – instead of focusing on the far more important qualitative differences – meaning sex differences in kind; different genes, different proteins, different circuits.

Ignoring these differences will continue to complicate drug development efforts. We know that our biology is different – there are tons of examples that show us exactly that. 'Wilful blindness to sex differences risks both over-generalizing findings made in male subjects and missing the opportunity to discover female-specific mechanisms.'

This gender pain gap also affects children and young people: young women are more likely to have their pain dismissed than young men. Things are even worse for black women, who are more likely than white women to have their pain dismissed and receive poorer pain treatment.

People believe that women are better at coping with pain, just because we suffer a lot of it as part of being a woman, with things like our periods and childbirth. All of this adds up to our pain being thought of as 'natural'.

But here's some exciting news. Professor Mychasiuk thinks that 'where we're going to make the most advancements the fastest is actually helping females. I don't know if you've come across this in your research, but 95 per cent of

---

[13] https://pubmed.ncbi.nlm.nih.gov/23165262/

all pain research has been done in middle-aged white dudes. And then for some reason we've only researched middle-aged male mice, middle-aged male rats – very little has been done in females.'

That's changing, and there is definitely some work in female mice and chronic pain, but as Professor Watt says, 'Just not enough and for long enough.' But studies are increasing since the requirement of many funding bodies includes consideration of sex in animal experiments. Though sadly a lot of this work in the USA is being shut down/having its funding withdrawn due to government policy on so-called 'politically correct' research around gender. This is super important given that the US has historically been the world leader in biomedical science.

Why does Professor Mychasiuk think researchers have avoided investigating women, or even using female rodents? 'Because no one wants to touch the oestrous cycle is definitely part of the reason.' That said, there are certain fields where the female monthly cycle is one of the biggest things that researchers are looking at, multiple sclerosis (MS) for example. We know that your risk for MS or the rate of degeneration in MS goes down if you have children and then it goes up at menopause. There are triggers that are definitely linked to females and their oestrus cycle across the lifespan. MS is an inflammatory autoimmune disease, too. 'Not that it would be definitely applicable, but this research would be able to inform a lot of other research to say, Hey, if it's happening in MS, it's probably happening in other things too,' she says.

Professor Mychasiuk adds, 'I would say there's a lot of hope because I think that they're easy fixes – if this drug doesn't work for women, but this one will because it acts on receptors that women have; we have a lot of that information, we just didn't look at the mechanisms before.'

I keep wanting to write how shocked I am at all this, but I'm not shocked. I'm a woman. I'm sadly quite used to this; mostly, I feel exhausted, let down and angry. Why are we only interested in women's bodies when we're critiquing or policing them? Why isn't there a funder curious to learn how our bodies are different from male bodies? It's encouraging that things are starting to change for the better a bit now; it really is about bloody time.

One researcher I spoke with is looking at part of that question. Fiona Watt is Clinical Associate Professor in Rheumatology and a UKRI Future Leaders Fellow at Imperial College London. In her clinic she noticed that many female patients in their fifties were presenting with osteoarthritis, so she's been researching what happens to women's joints during menopause. One of the questions she's been looking at is could menopause, with its lack of key hormones, be contributing to or even causing arthritis in these patients?

It's important to note the difference between HRT (hormone replacement therapy) and the hormones we have before menopause: HRT isn't exactly what we have before menopause. It's a replacement; it doesn't put everything back to the way it was before. It doesn't include all the hormones that you lose, and there's often a gap. 'It's not a straightforward question because "once the door is open, can you shut it again?" is a really, really important question,' Professor Watt says.

What happens in menopause that could increase pain? It could increase the tendency towards conditions like arthritis, or it could make them worse. 'If we think about sex hormones when they're there and what they're doing, that can be quite helpful. We often think about oestrogen, but I think it's really important to think about progesterone and testosterone as other really important players,' she says.

These hormones can modulate the pain experience, and they do this from the brain all the way down to our nerves, as they feed down to the spinal cord, to our peripheral nerves. They will modulate pain at each level. It's a massively complex system and there are things within it, such as pregnancy, where there are different hormones at play and where the pain we experience can be quite different.

When she mentions pregnancy, I tell her that I've been told if I ever became pregnant, I would experience remission of my symptoms. So what's going on in pregnancy that's so magical?

Professor Watt thinks oestrogen is the answer, and it seems to be doing two different things. 'We know that oestrogen can be anti-inflammatory. There's quite a lot of data showing that it can interfere with your immune system to turn down pro-inflammatory signals and promote reparative signals,' she says. Researchers have known about this anti-inflammatory effect of oestrogen for a while. And as you start to lose oestrogen, you may have more of the cytokines and molecules floating around that stoke inflammation, which turns up the volume on inflammatory processes and, of course, pain.

A lot of those molecules are pro-nociceptive or pro-pain molecules, such as IL6 or TNF alpha, which you may be familiar with if, like me, you take biologics to treat your arthritis, because these are the molecules our drugs target. In perimenopause and post-menopause we end up with an environment where we may be more susceptible to inflammation – which sounds bad, but there might also be some benefits. For instance, it's easier to deal with bugs with some of these things floating around, but in a pain setting that's probably not a good thing.

But it's not just our pain that can increase. 'I think your connective tissues also suffer as we go into menopause,' Professor Watt says. With osteoporosis, as we lose oestrogen, we lose bone density because the bone is very oestrogen-sensitive. But that's not exclusive to bone. There are oestrogen receptors and testosterone receptors on articular cartilage, on tendons, probably on synovium as well. (Synovium is connective tissue that lines the inside of the joint capsule, and that's a bubble-like structure that surrounds joints.)

To relieve pain, as well as considering hormone replacement therapy, physical activity, vitamin D and calcium intake are key. 'All of those things are really important for our musculoskeletal health,' Professor Watt says. And they all play a role in maintaining joint health and in disease processes – which means that what's going on in a joint might drive pain.

The other really key thing is sleep. 'I don't know that people talk about this enough, but I am a big believer as a rheumatologist who sits in clinics seeing people that sleep is really fundamental to how pain starts, is managed and gets better. If we can actually help people to sleep better then their pain often improves. When we ask people (because we generally don't ask people enough), you know, 60 to 70 per cent of our patients in the osteoarthritis clinics have significant sleep disturbance. It's just we don't talk to them about it,' Professor Watt tells me.

What's that got to do with hormones? It's well known that perimenopause and menopausal women sleep worse so it's probably not an enormous jump to think that their pain might be worse. Professor Watt saw this a lot in a study she and her team did. 'One of the really interesting things was that we were the first people to say, "Let's not worry about menopausal symptoms, we want a menopausal group." For the trial, we need people who can take HRT safely so they have to be in the right age group. They have to be within one and ten years after their last period and don't have exclusionary medical conditions. We just need them to have painful hand osteoarthritis because that's what we're interested in, so we didn't require any menopausal symptoms,' she says.

Despite that, when researchers looked at the menopause questionnaires, all participants had very significant amounts of menopausal symptoms. This could be, for example, because people with bad menopause symptoms have more painful arthritis or vice versa, or it could be that painful arthritis is part of a broader menopausal syndrome. What researchers really picked up on, though, was that the pain was often in the context of poor sleep and other menopausal symptoms that disturb people's quality of life.

Professor Watt thinks there are four big pillars that make menopause a really important thing for people with musculoskeletal disease: pain modulation; inflammation modulation; connective tissue health; sleep and well-being. Why?

Because, as she wrote in a review of this area in a paper in 2018, 'Chronic musculoskeletal pain represents an enormous health burden, affecting over 50% of adult populations. Common sites of pain are the spine, knee, hand, hip and shoulder. There is a female preponderance irrespective of the cause of the pain. At the time of menopause, musculoskeletal pain is reported by more than half of women. Presentation with joint pain in women is greatest between 45 and 55 years of age. Although this appears to implicate the menopause and estrogen deficiency, direct causal evidence of a role for menopause is lacking, partly because musculoskeletal pain is so common throughout life. Women are approximately twice as likely to have joint pain and stiffness around the time or after the menopause than their premenopausal counterparts, when adjusted for age. However, many such epidemiological studies do not differentiate musculoskeletal pain from arthritis, so assessing the burden of arthralgia [joint pain] and arthritis in these populations is difficult.'[14]

Musculoskeletal (MSK) pain, under NICE guidance,[15] can be considered as part of thinking about HRT because musculoskeletal pain, whether that's joint pain or muscle pain, can be considered as part of the constellation of menopausal

---

[14] https://journals.sagepub.com/doi/10.1177/2053369118757537

[15] https://www.nice.org.uk/guidance/ng23

symptoms. Her point is that menopause isn't only the symptoms we think of easily – sleep disturbances, mood swings, brain fog, feeling rubbish – it's also musculoskeletal symptoms. 'Map them. Record them. Don't change lots of other things, because otherwise we won't know what's made them better,' she says. 'So don't start your new biologic on the Tuesday and HRT on the Wednesday because I won't be able to tell you which has made you feel terrific.'

Would someone with musculoskeletal pain need or benefit from HRT along with their regular pain and disease treatments? 'I absolutely do not sit there and say you should take this for your arthritis, because we just lack the evidence for it at the moment,' Professor Watt says. There's a lot we need to understand about HRT. For example, if people start on HRT and then suddenly stop it – they'll present with hand osteoarthritis within a few months of stopping it. 'I think the reason for this sudden onset might be because stopping HRT overnight is inducing this completely non physiological situation, and although someone might have been having some problems with it, it's probably been doing some other things,' she says. In a recent study, Professor Watt withdrew HRT over four weeks from women with painful hand osteoarthritis who had been taking it as part of a trial. She thought it was a fairly cautious timeline, but the results were surprising.

'We saw far more people flaring with their pain when withdrawing in the active arm (from HRT) than we did on the placebo arm,' Professor Watt tells me. One of the things she tells her patients who are taking HRT is that, unless there's a real safety issue, do not stop this quickly. Stop it super slowly – months or even years. 'Because otherwise we end up creating an additional problem for people who feel even worse because they've come off it quickly.' She's keen that people don't get the wrong message. 'HRT is very good for lots of different things, but we have to be clear what it's doing and when it should be used in the context of arthritis,' she says.

Her interest in menopause and rheumatology was driven by the fact that she sees a lot of postmenopausal women in her clinic. The biggest problem is that people just don't talk about menopause in the context of their pain, and doctors don't link the two, so they don't see a woman in the clinic and question what else is going on here. How could menopause be affecting pain or quality of life? 'I think this is not a conversation that's had enough,' she says.

Much as I love my rheumatology team, no one's ever asked about any menopausal symptoms I might have been having. She finds it 'quite flabbergasting' that across the board in rheumatology, nearly all of the other autoimmune diseases, things like rheumatoid and osteoarthritis, have a massive female preponderance. But in 2025 we haven't even scratched the surface of why this is so different and why this is the case for so many musculoskeletal conditions.

'I think sex hormones are part of it and for me a lot of this is about why, for a lot of these conditions, they suddenly get a lot more prevalent after 50, you know? Osteoarthritis is one, rheumatoid arthritis is probably another,' she says. There are some women developing lupus, developing fibromyalgia, developing rheumatoid in that earlier, pre-50, age group.

'I think we know very little about that', she says. 'There's just this huge gap, which frustrates me enormously. We're just looking at one little bit of the elephant, but I'm sure there are some other other bits as well that probably aren't just about sex hormones, but that's the thing that changes, isn't it? But I suppose it's also their effects on tissues as well.'

Professor Watt points out that a big question we should be asking is how much do we measure menopause? How much do doctors pick up on it in the clinic when they're not being asked to look at it in the context of other conditions? What is normal? Normal is a median age of 50 to 51, but the NHS would say 45 onwards, but from 40 to 45, you're a bit early for menopause. At 40 you'd be in premature ovarian insufficiency. The question might then become: how does autoimmunity nuance those changes.

Could autoimmune disease influence our bodies in terms of having a lower baseline of protective sex hormones? Oestrogen is produced by functioning ovarian follicles that go through their usual cycle, 'so I think anything that would affect ovarian function would then have a knock-on effect on sex hormones,' Professor Watt says. 'You're raising an interesting question. We have a lot of tissues that produce oestrogen and that becomes a very important source of oestrogen after menopause. But the answer is, I don't know.'

Remember how we've seen that some drugs work for women that don't work for men and vice versa; what role do our hormones have to play in that, if any? There are some pre-clinical sources of mouse modelling studies that are done in forms of arthritis that do tend to suggest that for any level of disease – and this is true in osteoarthritis – female mice are often more sensitive and more likely to display pain than their male counterparts.

She points out that there may be some biological reasons, measurable differences, in the way men and women experience pain. I think of previous researchers we've met who've talked about how pain is socialised, how women are more allowed by society to experience and acknowledge pain (though, ironically, struggle more to have their pain treated). And how sometimes it's easier – or more acceptable – to complain of pain or seek treatment for pain, instead of something else, like trauma. That, too, is of course about gender roles and stereotyping, all of which are socialised into us.

'Pain behaviour is driven by a lot of things: the modulation of pathways, the inflammation being different and potentially influenced by the menstrual cycle, and obviously that's difficult to see,' Professor Watt says. 'Humans are very different to mice in that regard. They're not always good models of human behaviour, particularly in relation to the female life course.'

But if our inflammation is influenced by our sex hormones, could that be why so many people I spoke to for this book noticed their pain started around the same time as they got their first periods? I noticed my first set of strange, random attacks around the same time that I got my first period – but the pain didn't really 'take' until later on.

Professor Watt says, 'I think this question about what makes females different starts early in life, and when you look at some chronic musculoskeletal pain, the time you start to see an excess in females, it seems to be around the teenage years.' And it seems to be at menarche (the start of menstruation) and afterwards that we start to see increased rates of fibromyalgia in girls, increased rates of pelvic pain in girls. There are other painful conditions that can be seen in the younger population, so it does seem that, as women develop that sex hormone axis, there is a higher tendency to pain.

'Whether that links into being more likely to develop a condition like ankylosing spondylitis feels quite different to me,' Professor Watt says. 'Because that's asking a different question, isn't it? Which is, What's happening to my immune state now, is that to do with sex hormone modulation? We really don't know.'

I ask, again, if people with autoimmune disease could maybe just have low baseline levels of sex hormones to start with. Professor Watt says, 'People are less likely to be prescribed HRT with these rheumatic conditions. I think there is an inequity there. Because there's a general conservativeness which may be quite right to say, "Gosh, we're worried about X or Y, so we can't let you have HRT." But actually if you look at the population in the rheumatology clinics there, I'm quite sure there will be lower proportions now of women taking these things as opposed to if you look at people bounding around without these conditions, who've gone to their GP and are now on oestrogen.' She readily admits she doesn't have the evidence to say any of this beyond her experience, which would be that there's lots of hesitancy for HRT if you're being seen for other conditions, particularly in a hospital or specialist setting, because hospital physicians are more conservative than GPs, and GPs would look to specialists to advise in this scenario.

There's also the challenge of getting new research into education and into the clinic that she mentions, and again, she's not the only researcher who suggests to me that there is a gap in the way new research – or even just established current knowledge about menopause and HRT – is shared with clinicians. Very often it feels as though clinicians are living with the data they grew up with at medical school or as junior doctors – which might be decades out of date – and then they've trained in their specialty and they've never interacted or thought about women's health, unless perhaps they are themselves menopausal women and then they may have some insight. 'But there's actually no cross-training,' she says. 'So as a rheumatologist, no one sends me on a course to learn about HRT or menopause. So lo and behold, no one tells clinicians that, actually, we've moved on and there are safer drugs, and that transdermal oestrogens are safer than taking it as a tablet.'

She thinks it's gradually changing, and that might be from increased public health awareness (thanks, Davina!) and the agenda that's now coming from the government around this. 'But it's certainly not coming from the general medical profession enough,' she says. She did a review recently, and at the end of it she said that women's health needs to talk to rheumatology and rheumatology for sure needs to talk to women's health. 'And we need to think about our conditions in each other's clinics. Whenever I stand up on a podium now about this, I also make that point, but that's a drop in the ocean,' Professor Watt says. It's not good enough. We need to get women's health into the postgraduate education agenda.

From her perspective, the main thing is for clinicians in all the specialties and GPs to have a bit of knowledge around menopause and HRT: 'It seems like it's so easy to say, "Oh well, this isn't my thing." But it needs to be because it affects such a large proportion of the patient population.'

WHAT'S THE CENTRAL NERVOUS SYSTEM GOT TO DO WITH IT? 5

When I meet Professor Marco Loggia, a neuroscientist at Harvard, he starts by telling me about his Canadian connections: he did his PhD at McGill (in Montreal), and he has the good fortune to have a Canadian wife, which I immediately congratulate him on.

Why did he start investigating pain? 'I was very interested and fascinated early on about the brain and neuroscience, in particular. I wanted to find a subfield of neuroscience that would have a strong clinical implication and connection with life,' he says. And in the past ten years that's brought him to study pain. His lab has focused mostly on understanding what the role of neuroinflammation is in chronic pain conditions.

His jurisdiction, if you will, initially focused on the brain and spinal cord, but more recently he's begun investigating inflammation across the entire body, beyond the nervous system to include things like our joints.

The nervous system has two main parts: the central nervous system (CNS), which is your brain and spinal cord; and your peripheral nervous system (PNS), which is a bunch of nerves all branching out from your spinal cord. Within this system is your somatic nervous system, which deals with your voluntary movements, and your autonomic nervous system, which is in charge of the things you do without thinking about.

Lots of conditions or disorders affect your nervous system, such as Alzheimer's disease, cancer, infections like meningitis, stroke.

Microglia are glial cells – and glial cells are the most common cells in the CNS. They contribute to the establishment or maintenance of persistent pain. We know that if you block these cells in animals, the pain responses are reduced. But can we do that in humans? That's the big question that Professor Loggia and his lab are trying to answer.

In 2015, Professor Loggia's team were the first to find evidence of neuroinflammation in key regions of the brains of patients with chronic pain. They showed levels of an inflammation-linked protein – called the translator protein (or TSPO) – are elevated in parts of the brain that are involved in pain transmission. This finding opens up new potential treatment strategies. But, more importantly, the study also gives researchers a way around one of the most frustrating challenges in chronic pain – that there's no way to objectively measure the presence or intensity of pain.

They saw elevated TSPO in the thalamus, which is the body's information relay station. All information from your body's senses (except smell) is processed through your thalamus before being sent to your brain's cerebral cortex for interpretation. Your thalamus also plays a role in sleep, wakefulness, consciousness, learning and memory.

Professor Loggia's team found that they could determine who had chronic back pain just by looking at the scans, because that signal was so elevated. And that's really rare – which made them pretty excited.

They did more studies and the big picture that's developing is that this signal, the translocator protein, has a different meaning in different parts of the brain. Researchers saw that people who have more nociplastic pain also have more of the signal in the primary somatosensory cortex (the part of your brain that processes sensations from the body, including pain). And they also found a clear association between the TSPO and depressive symptoms in parts of the brain that are involved in emotional processing. 'Unfortunately, there's a lot of comorbidity between pain and depression,' Professor Loggia says. 'Of course, if you have pain, you know – sometimes it's tough, right?'

Next, his research team looked at the spinal cord. 'The brain is easier to image, because as long as people lie still in the scanner, it doesn't move. It is also quite large. The spinal cord is pretty tricky because it's smaller, and it fluctuates every time your heart beats. But even in the spinal cord, in patients with pinched nerves in their lumbar spine, we found a higher signal.

'This was exciting. We thought we'd just got lucky, that we chose the only condition that has this kind of feature. Because this can't be true, right? But we decided to test it some more, and we started looking elsewhere, and wherever we look, we're finding it.'

They've published a paper showing TSPO elevation is very widespread in the brain of patients with fibromyalgia, and they're seeing similar patterns in veterans with Gulf War Syndrome, which refers to the unexplained illnesses occurring in veterans of the 1991 Gulf War. It isn't well understood, but clinically it presents similar to fibromyalgia, with symptoms like widespread pain, non-refreshing sleep and difficulty concentrating. They also found elevated TSPO signal in migraine, so it seems to be a widespread and pervasive phenomenon.

All of this is great and exciting news, but, as Professor Loggia says, 'Now we have to figure out what does it all mean, and can we do anything about it?' I ask if it could it mean that this TSPO marker is potentially a druggable target? As in, could we make a drug that would go after this TSPO and switch off our pain?

'I can give you two answers,' Professor Loggia says. 'So yes, I think that there are drugs that can be used, but it's unclear whether you want to inhibit expression of this protein, or actually you want to use agonists, right? People suggest that TSPO is up-regulating in the context of an inflammatory response – so, when you see inflammation, it goes up. However, some think that maybe it acts as a brake, maybe it acts as a negative regulator of inflammation.' Maybe what researchers are imaging are the immune cells in the brain trying to quiet down the inflammation. But the jury's still out. 'To me, the big value of this is that if we're imaging what we think we are, then this suggests that targeting glial cells and immune cells would be a fruitful strategy, right?' he says.

The fact that TSPO is so widespread and they're seeing so much of it in all these patients, leads Professor Loggia to believe that it 'has to be something that has some importance'.

His team has also worked on studies with patients with neurogenetic disorders such as ALS, multiple sclerosis and Huntington's disease, and these patients all show some degree of inflammation, but the spatial distribution is very different. Which makes Professor Loggia think that the mechanisms are also very different. 'Why do we see the TSPO signal in the thalamus right in the middle of the brain, or even in the cortex? With that back pain, I think, and we don't know this for sure, but I suspect that what we're seeing is a response to aberrant, altered neural activity,' he says.

I ask him if he imagines that at some point in the future, if I go to the doctor for a bad back, they're going to treat my brain instead. 'Yes, I think that's a possibility. I think that's where we're going. I think that's where we're going because chronic pain is increasingly understood as a disorder of the central nervous system.'

It makes total sense if you think about it like this, as Professor Loggia suggests. 'Think about someone with knee arthritis – there are people who walk around with knees in terrible shape, bone on bone. Some of them even go skiing! And you also have the reverse, people with knees that are perfectly fine, but they need a stick just to walk.' The fact that a bad knee doesn't seem to predict someone's pain very well suggests that the pain might be driven by the central nervous system.

'This is kind of working model we have. At some point, you image the joints, or you image the back, and that doesn't tell you much, it doesn't really tell you how bad a person feels because it's their brain,' Professor Loggia says.

His lab is trying to figure out if the protein, that signal, can be used to predict development of pain. They've been studying patients with knee arthritis prior to total knee replacement – and this is important because it's estimated that 20 to 30 per cent of people develop persistent post-surgical pain.

So is it possible to do a scan to know the pain state of your brain prior to a surgery – and can that tell doctors if you're going to do well or not? 'That's what we are seeing. The signal in the brain actually has some predictive power – it can give me some information about those who will develop surgical pain and those who don't. If you think about it, it makes sense, right? If we see there is something that changes in your brain, well, I can replace all the joints you want but the problem is no longer there, the problem is here,' he says, pointing to his head.

The next big thing for the researchers is to develop a whole-person approach to inflammation – so instead of just treating the inflamed joints, there is also some consideration given to the brain. And if they can get all the information needed across the entire person, will that help to better predict post-surgical pain?

'I'm an advocate for the holistic study of pain,' Professor Loggia says. In the past few decades, there have been two important transitions. One is that we're moving more and more towards the nervous system and the brain, in chronic pain. The other is that we're moving from a neurocentric view to a neuro-immune-centric one. This is about integration, not looking exclusively at one certain part of the body, but looking at the entire person including the brain and the neurological immune system.

Professor Ted Price, School of Behavioural and Brain Sciences, University of Texas at Dallas, is also looking at pain through the lens of the peripheral nervous system, but he's got a really unique approach: 'I used to mostly do animal research, but I've stopped. We have a unique area of work where we work with the human peripheral nervous system and increasingly also with spinal cords by doing either recoveries from organ donors or by working with surgeons that remove part of the nervous system during the surgery.'

There are a couple of different surgeries where he can collect usable organs and human tissue, like a thoracic vertebrectomy. It's a surgery that people really only have because their cancer has spread to their vertebrae. Surgeons essentially rebuild part of the patient's spinal column, and when the hardware is put in, the dorsal root ganglia (DRG) is in the way. The DRG is a bundle of nerves in the spine that transmits sensory and pain signals to the brain. Each spinal nerve has a pair of dorsal root ganglia lateral to the spinal cord. There are 62 DRGs in the human body, forming 31 paired sets – one right and one left – along the spinal cord.

This cancer surgery is done more often at MD Anderson (in Texas) than anywhere else because it's one of the absolute best – if not the best – cancer centres in the entire world.

Patients come from all over the world to have really advanced cancers treated. That's important for Professor Price's work because these are pretty complicated patients, and they'll have pain on one side of their body and not the other, which gives Professor Price and his colleagues the chance to do detailed human studies on the DRG. They can compare one side with pain to the other side that doesn't have pain to discover what those critical differences may be.

'When people have chronic pain, in particular neuropathic pain, it's often localised somewhere, not all over their body. If you can figure out which DRG to put a local anaesthetic on, you can typically alleviate their pain, at least for some period of time,' Professor Price says. Sometimes, though, people will have so many levels of their spine that are affected that it's not really practical to do that, and it's not risk free – if you use too much local anaesthetic, it can effect the cardiovascular system, among other things.

The point is that by studying these DRGs, Professor Price and his lab can get 'pretty amazing detail' about what the underlying causes of the neuropathy and the neuropathic pain are in these people. They're using really innovative, leading edge sequencing technology to look with amazing spatial precision at the transcriptome of cells. A transcriptome is a collection of all the gene readouts present in a cell.[1]

By collecting and comparing transcriptomes of different types of cells, researchers deepen our understanding of what

[1] https://www.genome.gov/about-genomics/fact-sheets/Transcriptome-Fact-Sheet

constitutes a specific cell type, how that type of cell normally functions, and how changes in the normal level of gene activity may reflect or contribute to disease. So, for instance, with Professor Price's research, if they have a DRG from somebody who has neuropathic pain, and they can compare it to somebody who doesn't, they can get a reasonably good idea of what is changing in the DRG that might be causing that person to have that neuropathic pain.

Which is what most labs have been doing, looking at one gene or one protein at a time – using rodent models of disease. What makes Price's work really interesting, innovative and unique is that they're looking at the actual disease in human tissue instead of in a model. Obviously, they can't get DRGs for everyone, but what's really opened things up is their work with organ transplant groups. In Texas, most people with a driver's licence are registered as organ donors, and if you become an organ donor, your family can consent to have your tissues used for research purposes. 'If I die and become an organ donor, I would love for people to use whatever they can to learn whatever they can. I don't have a need for it anymore,' Professor Price says.

Professor Price's team have done almost 400 recoveries from organ donors at this point; about 20 per cent of the recoveries have diabetes and about 10 per cent of those have painful diabetic neuropathy. These organ donations have led to the development of an amazing data set on diabetic neuropathy, and the research findings are totally different than what was previously imagined based on what people have seen in animal models.

But animal models of diabetes are just that: models. They have a lot of use, but we may be at the edge of what we can learn from them. There's no real way to make the neural circuits of a mouse more like those of a human, and there's no way to make a mouse an upright creature that walks on two legs. We have low back pain in part because of the strain that's placed on our discs by standing upright, so how can a mouse model really represent the human experience?

Take diabetes, for another example. Most animal models use type 1 diabetes, but almost every person who gets diabetes later in life has type 2, and most people with diabetic neuropathy have type 2 diabetes. There are rodent models of type 2 diabetes, but researchers are artificially feeding the animal food it wouldn't normally want to eat or the animal has a specific kind of genetic disposition to being obese – it's just not the same as what happens in people. 'It's not even clear if rodents have pain in the same way that humans have pain,' he says.

Which isn't at all to disparage rodent models – they've gotten us pretty far. But to really make the kind of transformational progress in pain studies that we need, Professor Price believes it's important to use human tissue: 'The reason we don't do animal models anymore is not because I don't think they're useful. They are useful. But I happen to be in a situation where we have a good opportunity to work with human tissue, so we've prioritised it over other things.'

What started him on this path was an early observation that the human peripheral nervous system has way more immune cells than the rodent immune system does. And that means there are a lot of opportunities for thinking about how to modulate the immune system to control the peripheral nervous system in humans – opportunities that might not be possible in animal models because those cells just aren't there. At least not in the same number and in the same way that they are in the human nervous system. 'I think it's a really exciting time to be doing this kind of work,' he says.

The goal of Price's team is to increase our fundamental understanding of the human peripheral nervous system and spinal cord. To do that, his lab is trying to identify targets to make drugs for, and then they do drug development and create spin-out companies to develop the drugs. (Spin-out companies are slightly different to start-ups, in that a spin-out will also have a minority shareholder which is quite often a university.) So far, they've spun out six companies and they have two drugs that are currently in clinical trials.

The first drug unfortunately failed in the Phase II clinical trial. But the second drug they're working on, which inhibits a type of enzyme called MNK, has promise. To give you an idea of how long this work takes, Professor Price has spent twenty years working on it, starting with animal models and progressing to human physiological studies using neurons taken from either surgeries or organ donors. After all this hard work, his lab has managed to develop a 'peripherally restricted inhibitor of these kinases', so that it doesn't get into the brain – it stays in the peripheral nervous system. They're nearing completion of Phase I clinical trials now – so, looking at safety, and then, if successful, they'll move on to efficacy trials.

Professor Price is rightly proud of his lab's work. 'I have high hopes for this,' he says. 'Basically, what we've shown is that cytokines and growth factors that increase the excitability of nociceptors – these pain-sensing neurons in the peripheral nervous system – they use this signalling pathway. It's an intracellular signalling pathway to increase the excitability of cells and basically it changes the gene expression so that they become more excitable. I'm convinced that fundamentally that's the underlying cause of neuropathic pain. And I think that this drug has a really good opportunity to have great efficacy for neuropathic pain and rheumatoid arthritis.' They'll know in about two to three years.[2]

It must be really gratifying to see the culmination of twenty years of research work. 'It's like a dream come true,' he says. 'I really mean that. The reason I did a PhD in pharmacology rather than neuroscience is because I wanted to be able to understand the process of developing drugs. And I got a really great education on that when I was doing my PhD and an even better education from actually working with medicinal chemists, like James Sahn (PhD), my partner in developing MNK inhibitors, and others who do this for a living.'

Professor Price is going to keep using human data from people with specific diseases because he thinks this will give them – and us – a much better foundation in how the

---

[2] We spoke in late 2024, so keep an eye on his lab's webpage for news: https://paincenter.utdallas.edu/

human nervous system works, and how to think about new targets and how to manipulate them. He believes this is an area that's expanding pretty dramatically: 'There's still a really good opportunity to develop small molecules that can potentially be efficacious for pain, and then there are other modalities like oligonucleotide-based technologies. I think with mRNA technology – as we've seen with vaccines – there's huge opportunity there to get better targeting mechanisms and to overcome some of the toxicity issues that people see with viral vectors.' So essentially developing drugs that target the mechanisms of pain better, and do so with fewer side effects.

It's great that Professor Price and his team are working towards developing new drugs. But what happens now? Over the course of my research for this book, and my first-hand experience, it seems like doctors aren't very good at accepting that there's nothing they can do and telling their patients as much, whereas researchers – at least the ones I've met – see these proverbial 'dark spots on the map' as an opportunity. This is almost certainly down to the difference of their jobs, but there seems to be a real reluctance on the part of clinicians to admit when they don't know something.

When I mention this to Professor Price, he agrees: 'I did my PhD at a medical school, and I know in medical school they don't actually teach physicians very much about pain, at least in the United States. And I think this is kind of well known now and also pretty problematic. When I'm teaching, one of the points that I try to make to the students is that as you progress in your professional career, one of the most important things that you can do is go from having this idea that humans actually know a lot of things, to the understanding that humans actually don't know very many things. Part of the great mystery of medicine is that there's not often a very clear answer to why people are having the symptoms that they have and that you really have to be able to try to think about solving the mystery. And understand that not every patient is going to be or suit the same answer either. But our tools are often built around some degree of sameness or uniformity. When we talk about pain and potentially a magic bullet to cure it, opioids might be the closest that we will ever get to that, but as anybody who has chronic pain knows, they're terrible. They don't work very well for chronic pain, if at all. So there will probably never be a magic bullet for pain,' he says.

Well, that's encouraging, isn't it? I don't think he intends to be depressing; I think he's trying to highlight the idea that chronic pain is massive, and comes in all shapes and sizes. And from what we've seen so far, there are so many potential contributing factors that something like a magic bullet would have to cover that it seems almost impossible. I mean, how are we going to treat a traumatic childhood that's led to a lifetime of chronic pain with a pill?

'I think that ultimately we have to understand all of these nitty gritty details, if we're truly going to understand how to help people with these pain problems that have affected humans, probably since our origin.' One of the things that Professor Price says is just getting going is sequencing: 'For the pain field, sequencing is just starting. You know, we started maybe seven or eight years ago in earnest doing this kind of work on tissues from people who have painful diseases. What I think this is going to do is to open up our understanding of the diversity of the causes of pain, and how we can get to the development of magic bullets for specific populations of pain patients.'

The paper 'Knowledge of the genetics of human pain gained over the last decade from next-generation sequencing' by Dario Kringel and Jörn Lötsch, published in *Pain* in April 2025, shows the game-changing nature of this work.[3] The paper explains how next-generation sequencing (NGS) technologies are high-speed, cost-effective technology to work out the order of DNA or RNA, which helps scientists understand how genes work, discover new genetic variations, and diagnose or treat diseases.

The paper highlights an NGS-based classifier that predicted extremely high opioid requirements with 80 per cent accuracy, highlighting the importance of tailoring opioid therapy based on genetic profiles. And, it showed that key genes such as GDF5, COL11A1 and TRPV1 have been linked to osteoarthritis risk and pain sensitivity, while HLA-DRB1, TNF and P2X7 play critical roles in inflammation and pain modulation in rheumatoid arthritis.

NGS has also played a role in developing innovative tools, such as a digital atlas of the somatosensory system in neuropathic pain called iPain. The somatosensory

---

[3] https://www.sciencedirect.com/science/article/pii/S1043661825000921#sec0165

systems monitor the temperature of the body, external objects and environment, and provide information about painful, itchy and tickling stimuli. The sensory information processed by the somatosensory systems travels along different anatomical pathways depending on the information carried. This atlas focuses on the dorsal root and trigeminal ganglia. The trigeminal nerve, also known as cranial nerve 5 or CN V, is a large, three-part nerve in the head that sends signals from the brain to parts of the face, and vice versa. We have two trigeminal nerves – one on each side of the face. They're one set of twelve cranial nerve pairs. The point is that this atlas makes it possible for scientists to analyse cellular changes during the development of chronic pain.

And here's something that is just totally wild: In a paper published in *Nature* in 2024, here's part of the abstract (like the blurb on the back of a book): 'Our research built and utilized the iPain single-cell atlas to study chronic pain progression in dorsal root and trigeminal ganglia. We discovered that senescence of a small subset of pain-sensing neurons may be a driver of chronic pain.'

In biology, senescence is a process by which a cell ages and permanently stops dividing but does not die. Over time, large numbers of old (or senescent) cells can build up in tissues throughout the body. It's not quite ageing – ageing is a process of progressive decline, but senescence happens throughout our lifetimes. There are several compounds for anti-ageing and cancer-related diseases that target senescence, so it doesn't seem like a big leap to think that these compounds could be repurposed to treat chronic pain and some headaches.

NGS is at the forefront of pain research, providing insights into the genetic basis of pain and paving the way for personalised treatment approaches. Ongoing studies have used NGS to identify genetic targets for novel pain therapies. For example, a clinical trial at the University of California, San Diego is using NGS technology to identify and treat potential urinary pathogens in female patients with chronic bladder pain and cystitis-like symptoms. And the National Institutes of Health (NIH) is exploring new models for testing pain treatments, including using NGS to better understand the genetic factors that contribute to pain. Always with the same goal in mind: newer, better treatments. Researchers at the Human PRECISION Pain Center at the University of Pennsylvania are using NGS to identify molecules or entire pathways that are altered in migraine, which could provide targets for new migraine drugs.

In January 2025, suzetrigine, an oral, non-opioid, highly selective Nav1.8 inhibitor, was approved by the FDA. It is indicated for the treatment of adults with moderate to severe acute pain. In the next five to ten years, NGS will likely reshape personalised pain management, particularly for chronic, cancer-related and post-surgical pain. The authors of the study 'anticipate improved biomarker identification, more targeted therapies, and enhanced pharmacogenomic applications'. The advances NGS brings will make more precise treatment possible and that has the huge potential for fewer and less miserable side effects. But widespread clinical use will have to get past cost and challenges around data interpretation, to name but a couple of potential obstacles.

'I'm totally convinced that the cures, so to speak, are going to come,' Professor Price says, and after reading more about NGS, I can see why he's convinced. 'We just have to get to the point where we actually understand what the underlying mechanisms are to be able to think about what the therapeutic should be. Maybe it should be a small molecule biologic, or maybe it should be a CAR T-cell therapy.'

Since he mentioned CAR T-cell therapy, what about my crazy idea to use CAR T-cell therapy to cure myself? 'We have our own ideas that we're exploring around T-cell modulation therapy. We published a paper on ICOS a couple years ago, which is a T-cell regulatory pathway, and the idea basically was to engage T cells. It's not that different from your idea around using CAR T-cell therapy,' he says. I try to remain calm and collected, which is extremely difficult because this sounds very exciting. 'ICOS is one of the pathways that people are looking at, and it seems like it has too much toxicity in humans, so I don't think that it can actually be engaged, but the principle is there. And we know that manipulating the immune system has really amazing opportunities for all kinds of ways to cure disease. I think that you can manipulate the immune system to teach sensory neurons to go back to the way they were, in much the same way that you can teach the immune system to start fighting a cancer rather than defending the cancer.'

Too much toxicity sounds like a great reason to walk away. But, as researchers keep telling me, science is about failure – you try something, it doesn't work and the fact that it doesn't work is actually good information. Knowing what doesn't work is another step closer to finding something that does.

Part of that work means collaborating closely with pharmaceutical companies, which has led him to believe that these companies are 'very dedicated to trying to find better therapeutics'. And that 'they also have come to the realisation that we're doing everything a little bit too broadly and we need to get more specific about understanding the mechanisms and then having targeted populations and clinical trials'. This would help researchers to overcome some of the key issues they're facing, like placebo effects, which are very real problems that need to get solved, 'if we're going to have a better chance of getting the relatively large number of therapeutics out there that people who suffer from chronic pain can use to get relief'.

From his perspective, it seems like the field is starting to move away from this idea of finding a better, safer opioid and towards very targeted types of therapeutics for specific types of chronic pain, like some of the NGS examples. There are already 'a lot of really good ideas that are moving into clinical trials now with the investment of the HEAL initiative at NIH, which has also played a big role'. The HEAL initiative is the 'helping to end addiction long-term' initiative, and it's a massive effort across all the NIH Institutes and Centres to accelerate research to stem the opioid public health crisis.

There's another trial that he mentions, which looks at a new treatment for patients with moderate-to-severe, neuropathic, chronic post-surgical pain and painful diabetic neuropathy. The researchers showed 'superior relief of chronic post-surgical pain after four weeks, though high placebo response rates may have prevented differentiation between their drug and the placebo'. But, still, as the researchers said in their paper, 'These findings are clinically relevant given that neuropathic pain is highly incapacitating, lacking effective treatments and representing a significant unmet medical need, and support further development of sigma-1 receptor antagonists for peripheral neuropathic pain.'[4]

'I'm hopeful that they'll be able to move those studies ahead,' Professor Price says. He also mentions psychological therapies that are being developed by a researcher named Tor Wager, who has developed a kind of pain-retraining programme. 'I think that's an incredible idea, actually, and I can imagine how it'd be very hard to kind of deliver that as broadly as what is needed,' Professor Price tells me.

Professor Price isn't just a brilliant pain researcher; he understands pain from an up-close, lived-experience perspective too: 'I think that it's really, really hard to live with pain. I had a spinal injury when I was in my thirties, when I was a postdoc. I was in really, really bad shape and got super lucky that my surgery totally fixed my problems. Before I had that surgery, the rest of my life might've been totally different than what I had planned because intellectually with neuropathic pain, I was a totally different person. I couldn't do it. I guess

[4] https://onlinelibrary.wiley.com/doi/full/10.1002/ejp.4755

I'm lucky in a way that I got to have that experience because it changed the way that I think about what I do.' That experience switched his thinking from just making discoveries to being very focused on developing therapeutics. 'My surgeons told me that it was kind of a coin flip whether the surgery was going to work or not,' he says. He needed surgery because of a major motor deficit and a paralysed leg. The surgery worked and he knows he was lucky. 'I know I wouldn't be the same person if the pain hadn't been cured. I also know that the available drugs didn't work because I tried. I had it long enough that I tried all the drugs and they did nothing. I definitely have empathy, and I know what it feels like to feel hopeless about it because I definitely did for a little while.

'I know some physicians don't take the position that giving hope is a really great thing to do. But I think hope is a fundamentally important thing to the human condition. And if you don't have hope, it's really hard to keep going.'

I'm so glad we have him fighting our corner.

THE BEGINNING, GENETICALLY SPEAKING

6

Where does our pain start? We've heard from researchers who think a lot of it has to do with what happens to us as children, but what about our genetics? What about the stuff we're given by our parents that makes us who we are, pain and all, so to speak? It's not a one or the other situation here, either – all these things come into play when our body manages to create the perfect conditions for us to experience chronic pain.

I get hold of Professor James Lee, Group Leader of the Lee Lab at the Francis Crick Institute. The Crick, as it's known, is an independent charity established to be a UK flagship for discovery research in biomedicine. It's a merger of the Medical Research Council's (MRC) National Institute for Medical Research and CRUK's London Research Institute. The institute was named after the UK scientist Francis Crick in recognition of his contributions to understanding the genetic code, the key to comprehending how living things work. It was established by six founding partner organisations: the MRC, Cancer

Research UK, Wellcome, UCL, Imperial College London and King's College London. What all of that means is that the government, two charities and three research-powerhouse universities fund it and the people who work there.

Professor Lee's lab studies how tiny differences in our DNA predispose us to autoimmune diseases such as Crohn's disease, rheumatoid arthritis and psoriasis. So what's wrong with my DNA, then? 'That's a good question, and it's a hard question to answer,' Professor Lee says.

Researchers know that for pretty much all common autoimmune diseases (like type 1 diabetes, inflammatory bowel disease, lupus and rheumatoid arthritis), they all have a really strong genetic component. Imagine firing a gun. Genetics loads the bullets into the gun, but then you need an environmental trigger to set off the whole process. You can have a loaded gun, but if you never pull the trigger it won't fire. If someone isn't genetically predisposed, then they're not going to develop an autoimmune disease.

At a population level researchers know that some people have evolved to have a hair trigger immune system – people like me, and maybe people like you, if you have an autoimmune disease. But why? When we evolve, it's generally to do something that makes it easier for us to survive. So what is this hair trigger immune system doing? Or what does it think it's doing to help us survive over the longer term?

Professor Lee gives me two great examples of this. He recently discovered a key role for a gene called ETS2. It controls the volume, or the activity, of a type of white blood cell called macrophages. A macrophage surrounds and kills microorganisms, removes dead cells and stimulates the action of other immune system cells. That gene seems to function like the volume control for a range of inflammatory diseases, like inflammatory bowel disease (IBD) and arthritis. 'We knew that there was a region of chromosome 21 where tiny changes in the DNA sequence could increase your risk of five different diseases, but what was really odd was that you would expect such DNA changes to be pretty rare in the population. Because if it's increasing your risk of lots of diseases over evolutionary time, you'd expect that to be selected out of the population because it's detrimental,' he says.

In fact, the ETS2 association is pretty common. Usually when you have something like this, it's common because the gene does something else. Professor Lee went to talk with Dr Pontus Skoglund, whose lab at the Crick uses ancient genomics to understand evolution and the human past. Professor Lee asked Dr Skoglund to use their data sets to see when this change in DNA first occurred in human history. For context, most of the changes that contribute to disease in people arose within the last ten thousand years. Dr Skoglund examined their data and realised that this particular DNA change actually arose at least half a million years ago, probably a million years ago.

That change has to be doing something else because a million years is plenty of time for something that isn't helping humans survive to be selected out of our DNA. Professor Lee's team discovered that ETS2 ramps up your inflammatory responses to bacteria, so before we had antibiotics, this would have helped protect from things like infections and sepsis.

Before antibiotics, this DNA change probably helped prevent bacterial infections from becoming established, which in turn might have prevented people dying. In fact, if you look in parts of the world where they have high rates of endemic bacterial infections, for example sub-Saharan Africa or South East Asia, the rate of carrying this particular genetic variant is not 70 or 75 per cent, as it is in Europeans; it's about 95 per cent. So almost everybody carries it.

'That may have been because it gave us a survival advantage if we were ever inoculated with bacteria, but of course now we've got antibiotics, and live in a much more sterile world compared to what people would have lived in before. This has left us with this immune system that's got an incredibly fine hair trigger,' Professor Lee says. 'We're now seeing huge increases in autoimmune diseases over the last fifty years or so. People have assumed that because the genetics hasn't changed in that time this must mean that environment is the most important thing, but I think that's a slightly simplistic interpretation.'

He thinks that while the environmental trigger is becoming much more frequent, the reason why not everyone has an autoimmune disease is that not everyone is genetically loaded for the development of these diseases. For those who are, it only takes a bit of a change in the environmental trigger to actually drive an actual change in the incidence of these diseases.

I'm really interested in the idea of an environmental trigger. I've always been told that, to the best of our knowledge, my disease was kicked off by something like having a really bad flu when I was a child. This sort of scans with my family history – my sister and I were both hospitalised for flu when we were little and we both have ankylosing spondylitis. My brother didn't get a bad flu like that and he doesn't have the disease.

But how do you look for that environmental factor or trigger? One approach is to use very large cohorts of first-degree relatives of IBD patients, thereby studying a group of people who are genetically loaded with risk factors. They're recruited at a time before they have any disease. Researchers then follow these people with regular sampling and questionnaires. And of those, some go on to develop IBD, in whom you have samples before, during and after the onset of the disease, and researchers look at what changes as the disease develops. The problem is that all of this is predicated on what researchers think they're likely to find.

We know that diet – and a westernised diet in particular – is very strongly linked to the development of autoimmune diseases in general, but it might not actually be the food. It might be the emulsifiers in the food, or it might be the fact that in a westernised a country with a westernised diet, you also have lots more antibiotics and stress and more obesity. So the trigger could be diet, or the emulsifiers in the diet, or what the diet does to the bugs in the gut, or it could be nothing to do with the diet, and the diet is just a proxy for something else that goes along with westernisation. Professor

Lee states the obvious: 'It's really hard to figure this out. But it's not impossible. There have been one or two notable success stories in recent years. One example is a study a few years ago linking the Epstein Barr virus – the glandular fever virus – to the onset of multiple sclerosis.'

But even if researchers do know what the environmental trigger is, it's not likely to be something that you can easily just stamp out altogether. For example, in IBD we know that there's a higher incidence after you get a gastrointestinal infection (GI). But you can't prevent people from ever getting a GI infection, and even if there was something we could do, would people actually do it?

Given how brutal IBD can be, it seems reasonable to assume people would do anything to avoid it, but people don't always do what you'd expect. We know that the NOD2 gene is a major risk factor for Crohn's. Researchers looked at first-degree relatives of IBD patients to see if they carried NOD2 or not. They only did this in people who smoked. We know smoking is a risk factor for Crohn's as well, and after having identified people who carried NOD2, researchers then gave them either standard smoking cessation advice or smoking cessation advice and also explained that if they didn't stop, they were genetically loaded for Crohn's, offering even more reason to stop. The bottom line was that there was no difference. Most people didn't stop despite knowing that they were at significantly greater risk.

Professor Lee thinks that the problem is when people haven't experienced diabetes or Crohn's, but are asked to make a big lifestyle change because they *could* get a disease.

If people don't have a good understanding of what it's like to have that disease – that lived, first-hand experience – telling them how to avoid it doesn't seem to make much of a difference.

I wonder if scientists and doctors get frustrated with the rest of us sometimes. They work really hard to figure out how to help us, and there we are, ignoring their good advice.

That hard work builds on what's come before – each new bit of information that's discovered is made possible by the bit that came before that. Professor Lee's work was possible, at least in part, because of what Professor Paul Wordsworth – who's recently retired – did over the course of his career.

Professor Wordsworth is a genetics researcher who studied HLA-B27 and its connection to ankylosing spondylitis. I hope that he might have a lead on a cellular target.

When he was a student, he studied under Professor Derek Brewerton, who was making some important discoveries about the HLA-B27 gene. Professor Brewerton also played a role in bringing together physical medicine and modern-day rheumatology into the single specialty of rheumatology, becoming the inaugural president of the then new fusion group the British Society for Rheumatology.

'And this was a very exciting time because it was really the first time that genetic studies really started in multifactorial diseases,' Professor Wordsworth says. 'A multitude of genetic markers had suddenly arrived on the scene with transplant antigens, the proteins that that we use for tissue-typing, and basically people took every disease that they could find and tried to work out whether they correlated in any way with the carriage of these particular proteins. And as some people came up trumps, others failed.'

And that first discovery of HLA-B27 with AS? 'It was a phenomenally strong association out of the blue in Professor Brewerton's study of 75 patients. This was the strongest genetic association with a polygenic disease found up to that point and probably actually ever since,' he says. It really was a milestone in genetic research: HLA-B27 is present in about 85 per cent of AS patients (compared with 8 per cent of the general population), though only a minority of those who carry the gene actually develop the disease.

In the late 1990s, Professor Wordsworth and his team conducted a twin study in the UK to investigate the role of genes in AS. The study showed that more than 90 per cent of the risk for developing AS is down to genetics. It didn't exclude an important role for environmental factors in triggering the disease, but suggested that any such factor was probably relatively common (the sort of thing that most of us might expect to encounter at some time in our lives). This research led to additional genome-wide association studies to identify more of the genetic factors that contribute to AS.

Genome-wide association studies (GWAS) are used to identify genomic variants that are statistically associated with an increased risk for a disease or a particular trait. So HLA-B27 and AS in this case, where the carriage of HLA-B27 increases the risk about sixty-fold compared to someone in the general population. To do a genome-wide association study, researchers use two groups of participants: people with the disease under study and ethnically similar people without the disease. Researchers take DNA samples from each participant. Then, each person's complete set of DNA, or genome, is purified from the blood or cells, placed on tiny silicon chips and scanned on automated laboratory machines. The machines quickly look at each participant's genome for selected markers of genetic variations, which are called single nucleotide polymorphisms, or SNPs (which are pronounced snips).

If certain genetic variations are found to be significantly more frequent in people with the disease, as compared to people without disease, then those variations are said to be 'associated' with the disease, but the associated variants might not directly cause the disease. They may just be 'tagging along' with other variants (perhaps in a neighbouring gene) that do cause the disease, sort of like guilt by association.

Professor Wordsworth's research on HLA-B27 and AS is foundational to our understanding of the genetic basis of autoimmune diseases. The HLA-B27 gene is one of the most studied genetic markers, but even with its strong correlation, it doesn't guarantee disease development.

I have HLA-B27 and I have AS, so what's wrong with my immune system, when did it decide to go bananas? The HLA-B27 molecule itself in part frames the immune system, and the vast array of foreign protein antigen receptors that develop within the T-cell and B-cell repertoire are shaped by the HLA molecules – so, for me, B27 will be one of these molecules. In combination with protein fragments that they will bind to, they will bind preferentially to particular fragments, and then the body will basically keep T cells, which have some capacity to bind to HLA molecules and proteins. So, I have a bunch of T cells that are designed to recognise bits of protein that they're likely to come up against in the wild. That's part of the answer.

My gut microbiome may play a very important part in framing that repertoire. 'And there is quite a nice body of work which is coming up now, suggesting that there may be particular T-cell receptor types that are found in in people with ankylosing spondylitis and related stuff,' Professor Wordsworth says. 'It does look as if there may be a particular receptor usage that's coming up in people with these groups of diseases.'

HLA-B27 isn't the only game in town for those of us who suffer with AS. Researchers are also looking at a gene called IL-23 (the IL stands for interleukin), which is strongly associated with AS in these studies. 'This was very obviously an interesting target,' Professor Wordsworth says. Obviously is doing a lot of heavy lifting, so he explains what he means in easier to understand terms. 'It's involved in host-tissue specific immune responses and leads to the production of a cytokine called IL-17, which is involved in helping tissues to overcome infections. And that understanding indirectly led to a biologic drug called secukinamab being fast-tracked to use for ankylosing spondylitis. It was being used in various diseases, or about to be used in trials, but ankylosing spondylitis would not have been the first disease on any pharmaceutical company's list simply because it's got a relatively low profile. And despite the fact that AS affects up to 1 in 200 people in western societies, I think people don't recognise just how much of a pain it can be and how dramatically it changes people's lives.'

The IL-23/IL-17 pathway plays a critical role in the initiation of our immune response to many infections. The production of IL-17, a signalling molecule, increases local inflammation in tissues like the gut and joint lining as the first line of defence against infection. The discovery of IL-23's involvement in AS was groundbreaking because it pointed to a new therapeutic target – one that could be blocked by a monoclonal antibody like secukinumab. Other important genes involved in AS have also been identified – for example, RUNX3, which affects the development of T cells (the same cells that are involved in the HLA-B27 mediated recognition of foreign proteins). These genetic findings can be used to guide drug development by investigating the regulation of the genes in immune cells.

I like to think of it this way: these genes are trying to get to their end destination, and it's the job of the drug to stop them. I picture it like a villain trying to find my house, and the drug has to stop the baddie before he gets there – so knowing the route he's going to take means I can plan where I'm going to stop him.

But, even though researchers find these genes that seem to have a little or a lot to do with our diseases, the vast majority of common diseases – so, diabetes, IBD, rheumatoid arthritis or AS, for example – are what's called polygenic. That means there are lots of ways in which multiple genes, probably hundreds of genes, could have an effect. Although that effect might appear to be small from the GWAS, it could eventually point the way to discovery of a treatment with potentially dramatic effect. So, carrying the IL23R variant may only increase the risk of AS by 5 per cent, but secukinumab will put more than 50 per cent of people with AS into remission.

Finally, you never know what you might find. One of the strongest initial associations that Professor Wordsworth's group found was with a small region on the short arm of chromosome 21. It increased the risk of AS by around 20 per cent but seemed to be a 'gene desert' – this region of the genome didn't appear to include any protein-coding genes. However, this region also contains the very same ETS2 gene that James Lee and his group at the Crick found to be very important in IBD.

'So that was actually the first GWAS hit on that region. Professor Lee's work is a really, really good example of how you can take a GWAS hit and take it through various stages of functional biology and to then identify drug targets. Anything that works for IBD arising from this genetic association is highly likely to be effective in AS as well,' Professor Wordsworth says.

> *In June 2024, researchers made a 'holy grail' discovery – a major driver of inflammatory bowel disease and several other immune disorders that affect the spine, liver and arteries, raising hopes for millions of people worldwide.*

Professor Lee's lab are the ones behind that very exciting headline. They use genetics to try to get a better understanding of diseases like inflammatory bowel disease, though they're not exclusively looking at IBD in the same way that Lee does in his clinic. 'In the lab, we work on regions of our DNA that not only increase your risk of IBD, but increase your risk of other diseases as well,' he says.

Without me even asking about the new markers he's found, he adds, 'And in fact, the ETS2 markers that we worked on are known to increase your risk of about five different inflammatory diseases, including ankylosing spondylitis and primary sclerosing cholangitis as well as both forms of IBD.' (Both forms of IBD are Crohn's disease and colitis.)

Researchers know that they don't really understand what goes wrong in diseases like IBD well enough – one of the best ways to see that is by looking at all the new drugs that are going into initial clinical trials. These are the drugs that pharmaceutical companies have invested a large amount of money in because they think one of them is going to be their next big blockbuster drug. But only about one in every ten of those actually ends up becoming an approved drug – and that figure has been true for around twenty years.

'When I started as a scientist,' Professor Lee says, 'we only knew of about three or four regions that increase your risk of getting Crohn's, for example. In IBD now we know over 400 regions. So we've got this amazing sort of road map of exactly where – in our DNA – things are going wrong to contribute to why people get these diseases. We've taken the approach that if we can figure out what's going on in these areas, it might give us new insights into why people get these diseases.'

While it's been relatively straightforward to find these regions – you just need lots of DNA samples from people with IBD and lots of controls – figuring out how they work it is much harder. And figuring out exactly how a single change in one of our six billion letters of DNA contributes to a disease? That's probably the multi-million dollar question.

What makes it difficult is partly because most of these changes are not actually within the coding sequence of genes, so most of them are what's called non-coding. A gene's coding sequence is kind of like the blueprint for an amino acid sequence that makes up the protein, and the protein is a molecule that does stuff like help the body grow, repair and function. There are several regions that are gene deserts.

'When you do a genetic study and you find hits or associations in regions where there are lots of genes where their function is well known, you can create a story about what might be going on there, even if you don't know it for sure. But when you find associations in regions that don't contain any genes, it's much harder to try and figure out what might be going on,' Professor Lee says.

For a few years now, that's what his lab's been working on – trying to understand what or how these gene deserts are doing. 'And it was this one study we recently did where we started on this particular gene defect, and you never really know what you're gonna find. Anything you do find is a little bit serendipitous because you could find something really important, or you might end up finding something that was already known. In this case, we found something really important that we ended up identifying in this region that has no genes in it, but actually it functions a bit like a volume control for one nearby gene,' he tells me.

This was the ETS2 gene. Its ability to control the volume of macrophages – or, to put it another way, to get the gene to release more and more cells – is really important for ankylosing spondylitis and IBD because they produce lots of the inflammatory chemicals that researchers try to block with the current best treatment.

So what Professor Lee ended up discovering was that this gene, ETS2, 'turns out to be the sort of master orchestrator of the inflammatory responses in these macrophages. So much so that you can take a resting macrophage, you can turn up ETS2 and that macrophage ends up looking just like it's come out of the gut of someone who's got Crohn's disease.' With just the one gene being turned up, you can basically switch on all the inflammatory processes.

Researchers have long suspected that there must be some sort of central regulator in these macrophages, but they've never known what it was and that's partly why lots of the drugs we currently use target individual inflammatory chemicals that the macrophage has produced.

For example, if, like me, you have arthritis, you'll be familiar with the (seemingly endless) battle to stop inflammation. We're trying to stop the inflammation because it's believed that this is where the pain stems from. There are lots of ways to do that, NSAIDs (for example aspirin, naproxen), steroids sometimes, and of course biologics which work to suppress specific parts of the immune system.

Anti-TNF is one of those biologics. You might take it if you have arthritis; it works for lots of people. But for some people blocking the TNF doesn't make them better, or it might make you better for a while but then it stops working, so then you need a different drug. 'What you end up with is patients hopping between biologics and finally they get a bit better. The idea is that if all of these chemicals are coming from these inflammatory macrophages, then if you could target the thing that's activating them in the first place, you could have a cascade effect where you could switch them all off,' Professor Lee says.

So, can we just turn the whole thing off? Is that what he means?

The short answer is no. 'You probably wouldn't want to switch them off; you'd only want to turn them down a bit so that you don't leave people too immunosuppressed,' Professor Lee says. But if there was a drug that did this, you might have a really good treatment, so it wouldn't matter if you're only going to respond to one biologic and not to the two or three. Because you'd be turning off the process. You'd be turning everything down and then you've got something that might be much more effective across the board for patients with diseases like Crohn's and ankylosing spondylitis.

What I really want to do is ask Professor Lee about my (sort of crazy) idea to use CAR T-cell therapy to try to develop a cure for ankylosing spondylitis. But I'm nervous. I know I'm not a scientist, and he's been so kind and generous speaking with me and not being too technical. I really want him to tell me he's busy working on a grant application to fund a clinical trial. I summon up my nerve and ask him if is ETS2 a potential target for CAR T-cell therapy on ankylosing spondylitis. His answer is probably not.

Why? There's something called the transcription factor which controls when and how genes are turned on or off in a cell. And it lives inside the nucleus of a cell. Basically, it's hidden. All my nice little CAR T-cell killers could be gathered around ready to strike, but they just wouldn't be able to see the enemy. They can't peek inside the windows of a cell, so to speak.

'You could imagine doing a CAR T-cell experiment where you target something on the macrophages. That would be a little bit more complicated than in lupus,' Professor Lee says. 'In lupus we are fairly confident that we know which cells are responsible for initiating the disease and can target these specifically with CAR T-cells. We have a reasonably good idea of where the disease starts. We know that there's production of these antibodies so we can use the CAR T-cells to target them. But in IBD and ankylosing spondylitis, it's more complicated because there isn't one single event that drives everything.' Plus, Professor Lee tells me that out of those first six patients in Germany that I was so excited about, well, as it turns out there's already a report that a patient has relapsed.

Remember when Professor Lee said that one in ten drugs actually gets approved? Well, if the drug you're making targets the pathways that are implicated by disease genetics, then your odds of making a drug that actually works get a lot better. 'Originally, we thought that you might get two or three times better,' Professor Lee says. 'But there have been more recent studies that suggest if you know the exact pathway, you might get five or six times better results, which means you could take that terrible 10 per cent success rate and turn it into something closer to 50 or 60 per cent.'

What that means is that ETS2 is really exciting because it targets pathways directly. Professor Lee and his team looked to see if their ETS2 had anything like an intrinsic off-switch (because if it did, they could have tried to design a small molecule that would target the off-switch), but their studies suggested that there wasn't anything in the ETS2 that was an obvious target.

Instead, they decided to do something else. They looked for any drugs – which were already approved for use – that might be doing something that regulates ETS2. If this was a gangster film, they'd be going after your family, not you.

They used a database which lists thousands of small molecules, and which also has a list of genes that change when you put drug X into cell Y. Professor Lee and his team searched through all those lists and found about thirty thousand potential hits. From that list, they worked out one or two drugs that were already approved for treatment of IBD.

But, more interestingly, they found that a class of drugs called MEK inhibitors looked promising. MEK inhibitors are small molecules that are approved for cancer treatment and neurofibromatosis, but they're not currently approved for anything inflammatory, and to the best of Professor Lee's knowledge no other research group has properly looked at them with an inflammatory disease in mind.

Professor Lee and his team thought, OK, let's see if a MEK inhibitor might switch off an inflammatory macrophage, and it seemed like it was doing it through the ETS2. His team were excited, but cautious. Things go well in the lab, but that's not the same as trying them in people. Their next step was to take biopsies from people with active inflammatory disease and try the MEK inhibitors on those. And sure enough, it worked.

'What that means is, at least in the lab, MEK inhibitors look like they could be a very effective treatment for IBD,' says Professor Lee. 'But the problem we have is that MEK inhibitors are only licensed for use in short bursts because they have side effects, and they have side effects because the thing that they're targeting actually has lots of important roles into other tissues.'

Right now, they're trying to modify the MEK inhibitor so that it only gets taken up by inflammatory macrophages and won't get taken up by any other cell. It's quite possible that drugs like MEK inhibitors might be effective for IBD or AS in doses considerably lower than those used in short bursts in cancer treatment, which would clearly reduce their toxicity.

Professor Lee and his team have a plan and are testing compounds they've made in the lab to see if they're as selective as they need to be – as in, they're a sniper that only works on those inflammatory macrophages – and if they are, then they've got something that they could fairly quickly go into clinical trials with.

He's pretty confident that if they could selectively target ETS2 inflammatory macrophages, that would work. 'Now, obviously a lot of work still needs to be done, so we're not ready for clinical trials just yet. But we have got some work in the lab specifically on this project and we're hoping to get there pretty quickly,' Professor Lee says.

How does that make him feel, as a researcher? 'It's crazy. We've been working on gene deserts for a while. The last project we did, which was on a T-cell specific gene desert, we got to the end and we figured out all the biology and it did tell us something interesting about why T cells go haywire in IBD, but it didn't lend itself to an obvious therapy because it was going to be too difficult to try and target.' That's the thing about science, though. Any new knowledge, even if it's not the thing you were hoping you'd learn, is still useful.

But for Professor Lee, he's not just interested in figuring out how things work just for the sake of it: 'I want something that at some point in the in the future, we'll be able to prescribe to the patients I look after and actually have a chance of making them better.' In his lab, he's not a stamp collector. 'We deliberately go after genetic associations that are what we call pleiotropic. If a single change can drive your risk of three or four, five or seven or eight or nine diseases, we know it's important. But the second thing is if you can figure out exactly what's going on, then you have a discovery that may well be applicable to lots of diseases, not just one or two.'

What could ETS2 help treat? 'We can say off the bat that we think that we can potentially drug the easiest two pathways. We would expect to represent a therapy that could work in IBD and could work in primary sclerosing cholangitis and psoriatic arthritis. And so we deliberately go after these pathways which from the outset we are expecting could provide potential therapeutic targets across a whole range of diseases,' Professor Lee says.

Not unsurprisingly, there's a lot of interest in ETS2 now, and a lot of companies are now specifically focusing on targets that are supported by disease genetics. 'I'm hoping the next wave of treatments not only will be much more effective, but are much more likely to end up being approved for patients, because theoretically they're not going to fail,' he says.

It's interesting to me that he's mentioned patients. Of course finding new treatments and helping sick people is the end goal of all this research, but sometimes, some researchers can give the impression that they're more interested in solving a puzzle.

'During my medical training I'd seen IBD patients on the ward and they were all young and they were all pretty sick. And when I would speak to my bosses at the time about why does this happen or why does that happen, most of the time, they said, "Well, we don't really know,"' he says. 'And it really resonated with me that there was this large population of patients who had this horrible disease and we just didn't really understand it well enough.'

I wanted to know how seeing patients in his clinic effects his work as a scientist. 'It is hugely useful in terms of informing what we do in the lab,' he says, 'because on a weekly basis I see patients who are living with these diseases and having all the problems. I don't need to be told that we need better therapies for IBD because I see it week in, week out. For patients who are on a biologic, when things aren't working and they have to change or increase the dose – I know that is a major issue and therefore it helps inform the work that we do.'

And working with patients can more directly inform the work they do, because Professor Lee can take biopsy samples from his patients at the Royal Free Hospital and his team can study those biopsy samples to see whether potential therapies might work. 'That's exactly what we did in the ETS2 paper. It works both ways. It's a huge motivator for the lab,' he adds. When their paper about ETS2 came out it 'blew up' on social media, and he put some of the comments people left up on the wall in the lab. A couple of those messages were: 'This gives us so much hope.' 'My child has awful chronic disease, and this made me cry happy tears.'

New therapies will also make Professor Lee's life a lot easier too: 'I'm not gonna have to worry about which biologic to start, or is the patient responding to this one, or do they need that one or which one do I give them. We might have something that's much more effective across the board in patients with IBD.'

I thanked Professor Lee profusely for his hard work in the lab. Even though his ETS2 isn't the game-changing cellular target I'm looking for, I get it. AS just isn't as common as other diseases and it makes sense to work on bigger ones – like IBD – first because more people will benefit, and there's a decent chance that if it works for IBD, it'll work for AS.

Sometimes it feels like AS is a niche disease. I've had it for almost thirty years now, and until this past year when I joined a Facebook group the only other person I'd ever met with AS was my sister. But it affects 1 in 200 people in the UK, making it more common than Parkinson's disease and multiple sclerosis combined. It's usually one of those 'but you don't look sick' diseases (unless your spine is fused and you're stuck looking at the floor). The reality is that if left untreated it causes severe pain, has a dramatic effect on quality of life, employment prospects and life expectancy.[1]

Despite all our advances, we still don't know why, exactly, some people's immune systems develop diseases like AS and others don't. I can't say I'm not discouraged, but I'm also not that surprised when you consider the amount of funding that chronic pain research gets. In 2021, the MRC announced a £16 million investment in 'research consortia and a data hub to advance chronic pain treatments'.[2] There was also a £24 million initiative to establish something called the Advanced Pain Discovery Platform, which is a research hub for people looking at pain.

Approximately 8 million adults report chronic pain that is moderate to severely disabling. It is estimated that 43 per cent of adults (just under 28 million people) currently live with a degree of chronic pain in the UK. Chronic pain

---

1 https://www.ncsem-em.org.uk/events/my-chronic-back-pain-axial-spondyloarthritis-and-ankylosing-spondylitis/

2 https://www.cambridgenetwork.co.uk/news/new-data-hub-and-research-chronic-pain

may affect up to 30 per cent of young adults of working age (18–39 year olds). That £16 million the MRC gave to support chronic pain treatments is 0.32 per cent of the total overall health spend.

The situation in the USA isn't much better. An article published in the journal *Pain* in 2023 said that chronic pain is one of the most common conditions in the US, with more than 50 million adults reporting pain daily or on most days. Recently pain medicine research has been getting more funding, but the majority of that is focused on opioids – use, misuse and addiction: 'In the United States, there continues to be a lack of access to federal funding agencies dedicated to research in interventional pain medicine, which has significant implications for the development of effective treatments for chronic pain.'[3]

Despite all this, there are brilliant researchers who are working desperately hard to better understand our diseases – what makes us hurt and why – and developing better treatments. They're doing all this alongside teaching responsibilities and admin work and committee work – and while also applying for funding to do research. Most research funding, in the UK anyhow, works in three- or four-year bursts. You apply for a grant, then you have three or four years to work on your research project, which is never enough time. As the end of that funding rolls around, you have to apply again for funding – and if you don't get the next round of

[3] https://pmc.ncbi.nlm.nih.gov/articles/PMC10239629/

funding, your research stops. You lose good people – early career researchers have particularly precarious lives because their salaries frequently come out of these grants. So maybe you get a great job in a lab at one university for four years, so you move there, and then at the end of that cycle, there's no more funding, so you have to apply to new labs and hope you can find essentially a new job.

And yet somehow, these driven, passionate researchers manage to make progress.

DID I GET THIS FROM MY PARENTS?

7

Whereas Professors Lee and Wordsworth are looking for genes that cause specific diseases, Dr Keira Johnston, Yale School of Medicine, is researching chronic pain as a complex disease trait. 'A complex disease trait just means complicated,' Dr Johnston tells me. 'It's a specific term in genetics. It's in contrast to what we call Mendelian diseases, where we have one gene, one disease. So something like Huntington's disease, that's a Mendelian disorder. And there are prescribed patterns of inheritance we can use to understand what's going on.'

She gives the example of Mendel's pea plants. Gregor Mendel was a Czech monk who used peas in breeding experiments in the 1850s and 60s. He published his ideas in 1866, just after Darwin published *On the Origin of Species* in 1859. Darwin had worked out that characteristics could be passed on, but he didn't get as far as genes or DNA. Mendel studied how pea plants inherited different characteristics. He bred red-flowered plants with ones that had white flowers, and all those offspring had red blooms. When he bred the red-flowered plants with each other, most of the offspring had red flowers, but some had white. This was because the allele for red flowers is dominant, and the allele for white flowers is recessive. If both plants carry the recessive white allele, there's a chance the offspring will be white.[1]

When we think about a complex trait it could be something like height, or something disease-related like blood pressure. We can think about psychiatric traits as being complex, too.

But with Mendelian disorders, it doesn't matter what your environment is – if you have the genes for Huntington's disease, you'll get Huntington's at some point. Whereas with height, there's the genetic influence – people tend to be of similar height to their parents. But people outgrow their parents, especially if they had really different nutritional environments growing up. The things that influence us, then, are genetics and the environment, and the interactions between those two things.

When we think about the genetics that contribute to a complex trait, it's a lot of small genetic variations with small effects individually, but altogether it can explain more and more variation in the final trait.

It's not easy to imagine, and I ask if it's sort of like having all the ingredients in a cake. But Dr Johnston gives me a much better analogy. A researcher named Dr Jehannine

[1] https://www.bbc.co.uk/bitesize/guides/z2296yc/revision/5#:~:text=Mendel studied the inheritance of,flowers, but some had white.

(J9) Austin, who is a professor in Psychiatry and Medical Genetics at University of British Columbia (Canada) and genetic counsellor, originally came up with this following analogy to try to help people understand how these things work.

You start your life off with a semi-empty jar with maybe a few rocks in the jar. That's your intrinsic genetic risk for something like major depression. As you go through your life, maybe you accumulate a few more rocks here and there from things like traumatic experiences and stress and all the kinds of stuff that life throws at you. Eventually, you have a certain amount of stuff in your jar and you reach this threshold where you have that disease. It's about how genetics and your environment interact, and you accumulate risk from different sources over time.

The way that Dr Johnston looks at pain in terms of as a complex disease trait is thinking that you can have chronic pain as a symptom of a lot of different chronic pain conditions; you can consider it in the context of a site on your body – for instance, if you have low back pain. But you can also think about chronic pain itself as a complex disease.

'This is about thinking across diagnostic boundaries, which is informed by a lot of different things,' Dr Johnston tells me. 'If I want to know about chronic pain, I need to consider chronic pain as a disease.'

A big part of what she does is GWAS, and part of that is about trying to find the genetic variation associated with her 'trait of interest' – which is chronic pain. But because she's not looking at defined diseases, she'll often have to hunt for the trait that she wants to look at, and a lot of what she uses is questionnaire-based data.

And that data? Researchers have plenty of complaints about it – it's messy, or it's not objective. 'But chronic pain is a highly subjective personal experience, so there's no way for us to objectively look at it,' she says.

She did a GWAS study a few years ago focused on multi-site chronic pain and her data came from a really sparse questionnaire about pain and chronic pain that UK Biobank research study participants were asked at baseline.

The UK Biobank, if you don't know, is a 'large-scale biomedical database and research resource that is enabling new scientific discoveries to be made that improve public health[2]'. Basically, it's a massive bunch of de-identified medical and genetic data from half a million volunteer participants. Researchers from anywhere in the world can use it, too.

What Dr Johnston found was that multi-site chronic pain is heritable. It had what's called SNP heritability. A SNP is a most common type of genetic variation, each one represents a difference in a single base in a strand of DNA.

The amount of variation in the trait that's due to these SNPs that Dr Johnston found was around 10 per cent, which sounds small, but that's on par with major depression SNP heritability. Multi-site chronic pain also shared significant genetic overlap with a range of other traits, including major depression, PTSD and rheumatoid arthritis. Dr Johnston

---

[2] https://www.ukbiobank.ac.uk/about-us/

separated chronic pain occurring all over the body using a zero to seven score. 'The idea was that maybe people who reported chronic pain all over the body, maybe they had something different going on,' she says.

And it was found that this wasn't the case. Dr Johnston put all these findings together and looked at them at gene level to highlight genes that might be of interest, like genes related to cell cycle neuroplasticity and different immune processes. This sort of thing lets researchers look at variants, and investigate if any of those are associated with changing gene expression in different tissues. That part of her analysis highlighted the cerebellum and a couple of other parts of the brain.

She found a lot of genetic variants of interest, which is interesting and valuable, 'but it's hard to think about the mechanisms of how chronic pain works just from a ton of SNPs, even at gene level – it's kind of tricky.' More importantly, she's interested in the functional impact of what she finds, which means she's keen on understanding how this stuff affects people in a practical way.

So what did she find? The genes that popped up were ones involved in oxidative stress, antiviral and pro-inflammatory cytokines – a lot of immune things, but not strictly autoimmune. She also found things like cardiac dysrhythmia or an abnormal or irregular heartbeat.

Her current focus is nocioplastic pain (this is the one that's got no tissue damage, and poor sleep, fatigue, cognitive issues). Related to that type of pain, there's a group of chronic pain conditions called chronic overlapping pain conditions.

These include a core of fibromyalgia, endometriosis, interstitial cystitis and other gynaecological chronic pain.

People tend to have two or three or more of these things all at once, so they overlap within the person. 'I was examining those and wondered if there was a shared factor between all of them,' Dr Johnston says. She wanted to build a model of what she thinks is the relationship between nocioplastic pain and any genes tied to this type of pain. To do that she'd need GWAS studies of chronic overlapping pain conditions, especially the gynaecological chronic pains like vulvodynia, dyspareunia and interstitial cystitis, 'but there were no GWAS available because no one had done them,' Dr Johnston said. 'So I did.'

Since women are more likely to experience chronic pain, it seems eminently sensible to do these studies. And it's not anywhere near as shocking as it ought to be that these female-only pains haven't been investigated yet. 'I'm also trying to do GWAS of these gynaecological chronic pain conditions. As a standalone, I think that's valuable, but also I want them to put into my nocioplastic pain analysis because it's missing these key traits,' she says. This goes back to what Professor Beggs was saying about how a lot of pre-clinical studies – so rodent models – were using only male mice and rats. We have to include these female-specific pains in research if we're going to understand chronic pain.

She's cross-referenced all these genetic traits with a big database called connectivity map – which sounds a lot like a cause and effect type of dictionary but for genes, cells and different drugs. This allows researchers to take the genes they're interested in – in Dr Johnston's case the ones she's found that are associated with chronic pain – and run them through the database looking for compounds that might be good candidates for repurposing, though she cautions me that she's a couple of steps away from that. Her results have brought up a lot of established analgesics as well as a ton of immune modulating drugs. 'Some really interesting pathways were suggested,' she says. Which means that there may be drugs we've already got that we could use on these conditions.

In one of Dr Johnston's research papers, she identified a total of 89 unique genes; and 18 of those were established drug targets (as in there are drugs that target them), 59 of those 89 genes were newly identified with multisite chronic pain. These results could inform treatment development, and the research has identified a number of promising leads.

Dr Johnston told me, 'The whole hope of my research is that even though I know it's not going to be immediately clinically useful, it contributes a really small puzzle piece. On top of all the basic science, on top of all the pharma research, maybe what I do will help to understand chronic pain, and then we can treat it better because right now we're really not.'

8 HOW YOUR PERCEPTION OF YOUR BODY ALTERS YOUR PAIN EXPERIENCE

Massieh Moayedi is the kind of guy you have the good fortune to run into in life now and again: warm, open, funny and super smart. Based at the University of Toronto's Faculty of Dentistry, he studies how pain goes from acute to chronic in children and adults, with the hope of understanding the risk factors for developing chronic pain and why people experience pain from an identical stimulus so differently from one another. He's looking at understanding the basic mechanisms of pain in general, but also reminds me of the perks of university life, which is that he's got one of those jobs where, 'We're lucky and we get to study whatever piques our interest.' Which is not to say that his work or that of any of the other researchers we're meeting is frivolous – quite the opposite. Being able to essentially follow their noses means that researchers can act on hunches and that can lead to incredible developments.

But why does pain pique Professor Moayedi's interest? 'When I was nineteen, I was diagnosed with orofacial cancer,' he says. 'I was really unlucky, it was rare, and just one of the many cells that produce saliva in the mouth became cancerous. I had my jaw resected and the first surgery led to a lot of pain. The second surgery, which was to rebuild my jaw, didn't go well either. And I developed chronic pain.'

He was driving from Ottawa to Toronto in Canada, and the CBC had a radio show called *The Culture of Pain*. This episode was on 'Pain in Canada', and they started talking about pain imaging. 'I thought, This is cool,' he says. 'By joining a lab that did pain imaging, I learned about pain and as I kept learning, my pain kind of just subsided. Through education and learning I learned to control it. It comes back when I'm stressed or overwhelmed or tired.' Just like the rest of us.

In the past, when researchers were trying to understand pain, they'd look at averages, which means that everything – such as how we measure pain and how we treat it – was based around averages. Everyone is the same. What pain researchers noticed is that actually there's a lot of variability in how people feel pain, and people at first attributed that to genetics, which isn't entirely true.

What researchers are doing now is trying to understand why there is so much diversity in pain. If you look at acute pain and you were to distil it to the most basic mechanisms that exist, you have the ascending input, which is nociception – the signal that's going in. Then you have the modulating signals and those can be changed based on your context, your psychology, your attention, your genetics, any factors you can imagine. Ultimately, pain can be summarised in these two systems. And what researchers are finding is that people who are more sensitive to pain typically have much stronger ascending input and much weaker descending inhibition, meaning that there is less of a feedback loop.

In your body, every system has a feedback loop. For example, with vision you blink your eyes so your brain doesn't get overwhelmed with light and sensory information. There are feedback loops that inhibit the signal, so they try to minimise the signal because you want to filter out the things that don't matter. You don't feel your shirt unless you think about wearing a shirt, because you're shifting attention to those signals – you're opening the gate to allow more signals in. The same is true for vision, for sound, for smell, for taste.

We get used to things, but not pain, and for good reason: you wouldn't think, Oh, my arm hurts, I won't think about it. Pain inherently grabs attention, it's an evolutionary alarm signal, and you want to pay attention to it – pain is giving you important information. You want to mitigate harm, and you want to stop it. At least as far as *acute* pain goes.

Our bodies have a natural painkilling system, with five main pain regulating molecules that we know of: GABA, serotonin, norepinephrine, opioids and cannabinoids. These are involved in regulating pain inputs, and they work at every level of neural access, including the skin, the spinal cord, the brainstem and in the brain. These signals go in, but then they get blocked or filtered at every level. So the pain signal has to be quite strong to make it past these filters. The exception, of course, is if you focus on the stimulus, then you're exerting top-down control, which allows you to select for stimuli and turn off the filters.

People who are more sensitive to pain have fewer filters, or less effective ones, so that pain signal goes in much stronger. If that's a lifelong thing, and those signals get stronger, then in neuroscience the saying goes: what fires together wires together. Which is to say this constant firing works to strengthen those signals.

'Your body wants to make things easy for itself. Instead of using a small road to carry that information to the brain inefficiently, it'll make the road bigger,' Professor Moayedi says. 'What researchers think is happening is that the nociceptive system becomes more sensitised.'

As part of that, there are also structural differences that take place, functional differences that facilitate the input of nociceptive input to the brain. 'If the descending modulatory circuit is dysfunctional or less effective, that balance is broken and that creates more sensitivity to pain. On the flip side, some people have really robust pain modulatory circuits,' he says.

But why? There are a lot of reasons why these things can happen, and one that Professor Moayedi's lab is researching is around early adverse events. 'A child who has undergone a lot of stressors in early life can actually set that child up for psychiatric disease or pain. I think it comes down to the insult. Your brain is vulnerable or is at risk, and when a major insult happens while you're developing then this is what you develop,' he explains. This is exactly what we've been hearing from other researchers.

For certain types of chronic pain, like knee osteoarthritis, you have an inflammatory disease that's affecting your knee;

it's not about how much you're at risk of this or that. You have an inflammatory disease, which is due to your immune system. The interesting question for Professor Moayedi is what caused your immune system to kick off? Why is it different to other people's? What's driving that?

I lean in, excited at the possibility that someone might actually know why my immune system is bananas. 'Do you know?' I ask.

'No,' he replies. 'But we're working on it.'

They're also working on how our body image affects our pain experience. Professor Moayedi is particularly interested in body image, which at first seems like a strange thing for a chronic pain researcher to focus on.

If a man, who believes he is the breadwinner of his family, is injured and therefore unable to work, that can affect his sense of self, and that sense of self can be really diminished by his understanding of what he could contribute. Because he is unable to work, he can't contribute as much, and that's part of his experience of pain. But the whole stereotype we have of being a man involves being the provider, the breadwinner – and keep in mind that pain shares some of the same brain real estate as depression. For women, there are other aspects of stereotypical, gendered beliefs, like being responsible for the household and their appearance, and these social constructs are all touched on when it comes to pain.

Take, for instance, women who undergo mastectomy for cancer, or for preventative reasons – 50 to 60 per cent of them develop post-mastectomy pain. That's a huge number of people in pain and something we don't generally hear about, primarily because that doesn't fit with the 'survivor narrative' that we have in society. Professor Moayedi believes that changes in body image drive changes in pain. Increases in negative body image increase pain, and decreases in these reduce pain: 'It's not very different than feeling sad, and pain hurts more, and feeling happy, and pain hurts less.'

What about how we perceive or think of pain? Professor Moayedi tells me about a study that looks at how pain and cognition interact. For some people, when they get a headache, for example, they can't go to work and can't do their job. 'But for other people, when they have a headache, they're able to use the pain as a motivator. We always thought that it was a distraction-based model – but that doesn't fit the example of people being more productive in pain,' he says.

But value was never included in these models – what value means here is what people find more important. Researchers wanted to find out what people valued more (or found more important): the task or the pain. To find out they did a monetary reward task with a complex task, and they found that the distractions are value-based. If you value pain more, you're going to focus on that. And, equally, if you value the task more, you're going to focus on the task – as in, you're going to power through. All of that is absolutely true – for men.[1] 'There's a massive sex difference here and it's only when we separated the responses that we saw no effect in females and a huge effect in males,' Professor Moayedi says.

---

1 https://pubmed.ncbi.nlm.nih.gov/40788275/

Does that mean our ability to focus can help us to override the pain signals? Maybe.

Professor Moayedi tells me that the key thing is the mind–body connections like meditation and yoga can really change how we feel pain. 'The reason for that, in my opinion,' Professor Moayedi says, 'goes back to the idea of a body image. When you have chronic pain, you're not getting the signals of your body in a passive way anymore, you're actively selecting for the signals that are potential threats much more than the average person, and you're amplifying those signals.' It goes back to the saying that 'if it fires together, it wires together', and he is keen to highlight that he doesn't want patients to feel like they are to blame for their pain.

The example he gives is absolutely wild. Dr Roger Newport is a world-leading expert in the field of multi-sensory integration and body illusions. His research focus is how the manipulation of sensory input – particularly vision, touch and position sense – can provide insight to how the brain creates and maintains a mental image of the body.

He developed this machine called 'The Mirage Device', and you put your hand into it and it creates a visual illusion. Dr Newport takes people with osteoarthritis in the hand and makes it look like their hand gets longer or shorter. In his study, people's pain dropped 40 points out of 100.

Bananas, right?

Dr Newport's work is focused on how manipulating sensory input can encourage the brain to 'perceive and experience the body in a completely different way'. He looked at how something called mirror therapy and size reduction illusions can reduce pain in complex regional pain syndrome type 1 (CRPS1) patients, the majority of whom have disturbed body representations, with some reporting their hand as larger than in reality and others describing parts of their hand as foreshortened. If the brain's misrepresentation of body parts contributes to pain, then manipulating the appearance of those body parts might be a useful tool in the reduction of pain.

Dr Newport's research group did a study with twenty people who suffered from osteoarthritis. None of the participants were pain-free on the day of testing and none had taken pain medication other than paracetamol. Participants reported their pain levels before and after they experienced stretching or shrinking of the painful and non-painful parts of their hand, as well as before and after enlarging or reducing the entire hand.

What did researchers find? Overall, it was extremely beneficial, on average halving the reported pain in 85 per cent of participants. The really interesting thing was that pain reduction only happened when the painful part of the hand was manipulated. There was no pain relief when manipulating the non-painful part or when enlarging or reducing the whole hand. For people who found seeing their hand stretched helped, the average reduction in pain was about 50 per cent. And the shrinking produced about a 45 per cent reduction in pain. 'Remarkably, illusory stretching or shrinking of the painful body part temporarily eliminated all pain in one-third of all participants and in 41% of those for whom the illusion was effective. Although not formally assessed, many participants spontaneously reported an increased range of movement following manipulation and most reported pain reduction before active movement was permitted. Many participants gave spontaneous verbal reports such as: "I can feel my whole body relaxing"; "My pain has completely gone"; and "I wasn't able to move like that before".'[2]

Researchers went on to say that the results didn't completely rule out placebo effects. But 'the initial results suggest that multi-sensory illusions are a useful avenue of research for the treatment of pain in osteoarthritis'.[3]

Another researcher, Dr Jenny Lewis, at the University of the West of England, did a similar trial, using a modified version of Dr Newport's illusions, and found that it was less effective in chronic regional pain syndrome but found, 'a consistent but small decrease in pain related to an increase of likingness of the body,' Dr Moayedi says. Her study showed that 'people with CRPS frequently report distorted subjective perceptions of their affected limb. Evidence of pain reduction when the affected limb is visually altered in size suggests that visual illusions targeting central processing could restore coherence of this disrupted limb representation. We hypothesised that using virtual reality that alters hand image to match the patient's desired hand appearance would improve body perception disturbance and pain.'

---

[2] https://academic.oup.com/rheumatology/article/50/12/2314/1789180

[3] https://academic.oup.com/rheumatology/article/50/12/2314/1789180?login=false

Essentially, researchers tricked the brain into thinking the patient's hand looked how they wanted it to look. And that reduced their pain.

Dr Moayedi explains, 'We have these negative feedback loops in the brain that are maintaining pain. And selecting for pain information and amplifying those signals. This goes back to Professor Noel's idea that patients remember that their pain was higher than it was and they focus on the worst part rather than the best part. We have a bias towards negative information. There's a lot of ways you can target that, but one way that's most effective is to learn to listen to the signals of your body and not react to them. Detach the emotion from them, and just let the signals come through. And that's what mindfulness meditation does. That's what yoga does. It forces you to reconnect to your body and pay attention to the signals as they are.'

Which is, of course, easier said than done. But our brains are pretty powerful, so when Professor Moayedi tells me about another researcher who's looking into something called peak alpha and that it could potentially be used as a predictor for chronic pain, I knew I had to speak with him.

9 PREDICTING PAIN

Brain waves are the electrical activity of the brain, characterised by different frequencies, with specific classes, such as alpha, beta, theta, that are associated with varying states of alertness, cognitive activity and sleep.

Professor David Seminowicz, in the Department of Medical Biophysics at the University of Western Ontario (Canada), was working with a colleague who was doing research in development and found that alpha was related to cognitive dysfunction in children with ADHD as compared to neurotypical children.

Professor Seminowicz and his team were doing functional MRI studies trying to understand that problem, and he wanted to move into the world of EEG (electroencephalogram, a test that measures electrical activity in the brain). So he began studying the model that his colleague had used for ADHD in pain models. Their study involved a cognitive task which people did while they were either in a pain-free state or in a prolonged ongoing pain state. 'And it's pretty painful. We're using a capsaicin heat pain model, so it's pretty intense, like five to six out of ten pain that we can maintain for up to ninety minutes or even longer if we wanted to,' he says.

Researchers in the Seminowicz lab noticed some differences in performance of the task, similar to what they were seeing in ADHD. That turned out to be the less interesting part of the story – because another collaborator came along and asked if Professor Seminowicz was familiar with the literature on peak alpha frequency.

Alpha is just a frequency band. It's alpha because it was the first band identified in EEG over a hundred years ago. And you can see it clearly on a live trace, simply by asking a person to close their eyes, which shows you occipital alpha. You start seeing a peak of the waves, in the range of eight to twelve Hertz typically. It's thought to be involved in sensory suppression, so that's why you see it with eyes closed versus open. When the eyes are open, you're taking in the world and you have activity in the back of your brain, so you have a lack of suppression. But as soon as you close your eyes, you have suppression.

Professor Seminowicz then did a study where researchers recorded people's peak alpha frequency, which you can do by having an EEG cap on. 'Ask participants to rest comfortably, eyes closed for three minutes and you can get their peak alpha frequency metric,' he says. It's 'really nice' as a biomarker because you could record it in a clinic; you don't need a fancy research set up, you'd just need to wear something that looks a lot like the strap on ski goggles.

'Jumping forward to where we are now, this biomarker is something that could be tested in the clinic when a person presents at very early stages of a condition. Or prior to undergoing a procedure that has a high incidence of developing persistent pain, such as thoracic surgery, for example,' Professor Seminowicz says. The idea is that this would be one more tool in the physician's tool belt.

People with a slow peak alpha frequency are in a higher risk group for developing postoperative pain. In that first study, researchers found that resting state peak alpha frequency correlated with the pain intensity. Then they did a larger study with over sixty healthy participants, performed twice over eight months in the same individuals, and showed that peak alpha frequency enables them to predict – with a high degree of certainty – who is likely to be a high-pain sensitive person.

'That was our best prediction – identifying those people who are likely to be high-pain sensitive, which is good from a biomarker perspective because we can identify those people most at risk,' he says. Professor Seminowicz and his research team went back to his original collaborator, who did a small thoracic surgery study and used their peak alpha frequency biomarker, and again, the results were really promising. 'It showed that we could identify the high pain sensitive individuals prior to them undergoing surgery. So we predicted their pain intensity following surgery, which was really promising,' Professor Seminowicz says. 'I think that the prevention thing is real and if we can get it, if we can stop pain before it starts, that's probably where this is going to have the biggest impact.'

A lot of his time is spent looking for mechanisms that link the cognitive dimension of pain to the subjective experience of pain, and severity of people's chronic pain. He's learned that peak alpha frequency can be modified by either neurofeedback or by simple things like specific frequencies within music. They've also discovered which brain circuits peak alpha frequency is actually associated with and, 'to our surprise but delight it seems that it's the cognitive networks,' he says. Which is good news because it means we have a bit more control over it.

He prefaces his research with something that I want to include for you in full here because it's so important to really make sure this message hits home: 'I say this really cautiously because I'm so sensitive to the idea – I don't want to ever put any kind of blame on somebody who suffers from chronic pain. On them not trying hard enough to put it out of their mind. I know I'd be terrible with chronic pain. It's my nightmare. When I suffer from pain, I am absolutely useless. So if I ever develop a chronic pain condition, I've got a good toolkit. I've got a good network of people that can support me. But generally, when I'm in pain, I will reach for whatever drugs will give me immediate relief. So I don't think there's anything exceptional about people who don't have chronic pain. I always like to make that very clear because it's easy to get the wrong message.'

Professor Seminowicz's research points to peak alpha frequency being related to cognitive flexibility, which is really good because that's modifiable. There are lots of potential interventions that could increase, either directly or indirectly, peak alpha frequency and, ultimately, help alleviate pain. But there's still a lot more research to be done.

The next steps for them and this work are clinical validation – which means making sure it works in the clinic, on real people, who are in pain. 'We just got funding to do this in real patients who have early diagnosis of TMD (tempomandibular disorder) or early symptom onset of TMD, and we're going to follow them and see if this is predictive of the duration and intensity of pain, and the development of persistent pain,' Professor Seminowicz says.

While it's great to be able to predict who is more likely to experience pain, he wants to focus on ways of directly helping more people. 'I got into pain research because I saw a need to help people with chronic pain. Prevention is certainly valuable, but we also want to find ways to develop new interventions or improve existing ones,' he says.

He's done some work on non-pharmacological interventions, for example a clinical trial on mindfulness meditation for migraine patients, which showed that mindfulness is an effective treatment.

Professor Seminowicz's lab took the standardised, eight-week prescribed course of mindfulness-based stress reduction, or MBSR, which is used for everything, and increased the standard treatment time by adding an additional eight weeks of training (specifically another four weeks, but spread over eight weeks). They also added some trauma-based and migraine-specific mindfulness, and they tested it as a preventative. The findings showed that just over half of their patients had a treatment response, which is a reduction of at least 50 per cent in number of headache days per month, compared to 26 per cent for the active control group that was given headache education and stress management techniques but no mindfulness. 'That puts it amongst the best of all preventive interventions for migraine. So these are big effects. And there were other associated improvements with it that aren't typically seen in drug studies, like big decreases in disability, improvements in mood and in other quality of life measures. We showed that it's at least partially mediated by improvements in sleep,' he says. 'To us, it all comes down to this idea of the relationship between cognition and pain.'

With mindfulness, he says that their study offered training over sixteen weeks, and they showed that continued practice is really important, which is, of course, hard to do for people with chronic pain – and more generally people with busy lives. So he's worked with other researchers on getting the mindfulness training down to thirty minutes a day for five days rather than weeks and weeks.

'I'm optimistic about new treatments, but I'm also realistic about them and we've tried an awful lot of things for an awful lot of chronic pain conditions and the general rule of any intervention, be it non-pharmacological or pharmacological, is – best case scenario – you get a 30 per cent reduction of pain in 30 per cent of the patients,' he says.

Because chronic pain is multidimensional, it needs a multi-pronged treatment approach, which is why interdisciplinary chronic pain clinics are so crucial. 'Once it's established, there really does seem to be some serious rewiring of the brain that we still don't have a complete picture of,' he says.

Recently they identified a brain region that's consistently activated in chronic pain patients which isn't activated in healthy people doing the same cognitive task. 'People with chronic pain are using more brain resources,' he says. This study looked at migraine, but they're extending this to other chronic pain conditions because they have the data that shows this region of the brain is connected to a circuit they think has the potential to be modified.

This is abnormal, bringing part of a pain network into the performance of a cognitive task. 'But the brain's been rewired such that these things are co-activated so frequently that now the brain can't distinguish between what's a cognitive-related area and what's a pain-related area,' Professor Seminowicz says. The rewiring is so extensive that it's a lot of work for potential interventions to undo. 'Our view is that for the vast majority of chronic pain conditions, there's a peripheral component, a spinal cord component along with brain stem and cortical components. But for non-pharmacological interventions especially we really focus on the brain systems as something that needs to be reversed to get back to a pain-free state.

'We're working from multiple angles, converging on a way to get improved, non-pharmacological interventions. I don't think there's a real silver bullet there, so we – slowly – have to figure out what's working for patients, what people like and will tolerate and how to optimise those things.'

We're talking about how long it's going to take to get new interventions into the clinic, which doesn't seem like it should be that difficult. There are so many people in pain, so of course clinicians are keen to treat them. But how do they learn about new treatments? Yes, clinicians read the relevant medical journals, but keep in mind how busy these people are already, just seeing patients. In England, doctors are currently required to complete eleven statutory and mandatory training courses every year. There's 'a slow trickle-up effect for translation from discovering something in the lab that can work, to when it's actually implemented as state-of-the-art in the clinic. And that's partly on us as researchers. We need to do better at knowledge translation and mobilisation, and the universities want us to, but there's little to no support for that,' he says.

One of the things he's doing to improve knowledge translation is to start a pain research group (called kNOw pain) at the university, and building a pain community there. They've got some good internal support, and now they're working on external support. They're trying to expand across Ontario, and across all of Canada eventually.

So how are researchers meant to reach out to the wider population? To the people in pain who don't happen to work at a university or spend their free time reading academic journals? There's a lot to compete with, from social media to old school media, politics, shopping, families, life. So Professor Seminowicz gives me an example and jokes, 'Are you saying that everyone with chronic low back pain hasn't read my 2011 *Journal of Neuroscience* paper on brain changes in chronic low back pain?'

That study was in the *LA Times*, so if you happened to have picked up a copy of the paper that day, you might have seen something about their work. They were in the media for a couple weeks, different venues, but then when it's gone, it's gone. So then that information doesn't make it out to the people like us, who are in pain and might take an interest in that study.

Their findings showed that pain-related brain anatomy and function changes can be reversed with effective treatment. The rewiring of our brains that our pain has done can be fixed. They also showed that there's evidence of a link between regional brain function and anatomy. One part of the brain which is part of the grey matter that plays a significant role in mental functions, memory, emotions and movement (several conditions including stroke, Parkinson's and Alzheimer's can affect your grey matter) was thinner and activated abnormally in patients before treatment; after treatment that same bit became thicker and functioned more as expected when they had to do a cognitive task. This is exactly what Professor Seminowicz was telling me about earlier. And that anxiety and depression are closely related to these changes.

Wouldn't you love to have heard about that at the time? I would have, because that kind of thing gives me so much hope – it reminds me that researchers are working hard to better understand how our bodies work.

10 CHRONIC PAIN ON A POPULATION-WIDE LEVEL

Pain is a really personal topic for many people, but there are researchers working to understand how chronic pain impacts people on a population-wide scale, because this can give us important information on prevalence and factors associated with the onset and persistence of chronic pain. These kinds of things can be used to inform how we're treated in clinic to limit the severity of the disease and minimise disability, among other things.

Professor Blair Smith, at the University of Dundee, fell into pain research by accident, but he's stayed there for over thirty years. His work has been mostly in epidemiology, the study of how diseases spread and occur in populations, aiming to understand their causes and find ways to prevent and control them. Epidemiology isn't about studying individual people with diseases, rather it's about understanding patterns of diseases within groups of people.

His research has been focused on defining conditions, and then working out how common they are and which groups of people are more or less likely to suffer pain, chronic pain generally or neuropathic pain. From there, his lab looks at factors that are either caused by or increase the risk of these conditions, with a view to identifying factors that 'we can intervene in or that at least make us more aware that there's a greater risk of adverse outcomes, so that we can take preventive action,' Professor Smith says.

Successful management of pain often only comes, he says, after there's an acceptance that the pain is there and a diagnosis has been confirmed. That's a lot to get through before you're able to manage pain successfully. Why is that? 'Chronic pain usually means that all attempts to cure it have been unsuccessful and what you are having to do now is live with it. You did not choose to have pain but despite all attempts to relieve it or lead a normal life and control it, it persists. Coming to terms with the fact that your pain has defied all attempts to cure it and is here to stay for a while is neither simple nor easy.' That's from a booklet that was co-written by patients and staff at the Royal United Hospital (Bath) pain clinic to help people understand chronic pain.

They go on to discuss the differences between what acceptance is and is not – and what that amounts to is that acceptance is an emotional task that's a bit like going through bereavement and grief. You come to terms with something that is senseless, confusing, undeserved, that you didn't choose.[1]

---

[1] https://www.ruh.nhs.uk/zz_content_include/services/clinics/pain_clinic/documents/Living_with_pain.pdf

The simplest way to describe this might be to say that acceptance is coming to terms with the idea that pain is a disease, in and of itself. This is a really simplistic way of looking at it, but that's the principle that Professor Smith works from.

But why do we need to accept our painful lot in life anyhow? 'Research shows that if you can support patients to accept pain rather than constantly looking for a cure, you get much better results with your biologics,' Professor Sengupta – Consultant Rheumatologist at the Royal National Hospital for Rheumatic Diseases, Bath (and, incidentally, my rheumatologist) – says. He tells me about a paper that looks at people with low pain acceptance and it found they were more likely to engage in catastrophic thinking and had greater depressive symptoms with a tendency toward somatisation (that's a process where psychological distress is expressed as physical symptoms).[2]

Catastrophic thinking, in chronic pain, is when you believe that the experienced pain will inevitably result in the worst-case scenario possible. An example would be to expect to have severe pain forever, even if your lower back pain was mild and being treated. Pain catastrophising has also been linked to the development and maintenance of chronic pain.

Recently, reports have indicated that there are problems with the term pain catastrophising. These critiques are coming from a range of different groups, including us chronics. These reports, which were highlighted in an article, 'Pain

---

[2] https://www.archives-pmr.org/article/S0003-9993(24)00260-0/abstract

Catastrophizing: Controversies, Misconceptions and Future Directions' in *The Journal of Pain*,[3] are saying that the term is being used as yet another way to dismiss 'the medical basis of complaints and to blame individuals with pain for their pain condition'. Some people have suggested that maybe changing the name will help, but – and this feels pretty obvious to me – some really smart academics led by researcher Michael Sullivan at McGill University in Montreal, Canada are pointing out that renaming isn't going to solve the problem. They recently published a paper where they argued that 'continued calls for changing or deleting the term pain catastrophizing will only divert attention away from some fundamental flaws in how individuals with pain conditions are assessed and treated. Some of these fundamental flaws have their roots in the inadequate training of health and allied health professionals in evidence-based models of pain, in the use of psychological assessment and intervention tools for the clinical management of pain, and in gender equity and antiracism.'[4]

They also add: 'The place of psychological interventions in the overall management of pain conditions has been to complement medical and physical approaches to the treatment of pain; psychological research on pain and psychological interventions for pain were never intended to imply that the medical basis of presenting pain conditions could be dismissed.'

[3] https://www.jpain.org/article/S1526-5900(23)00471-6/fulltext

[4] https://www.jpain.org/action/showPdf?pii=S1526-5900(23)00471-6

There is a lot more work that needs to be done beyond changing the name, and in the paper, researchers suggest healthcare professionals get up-to-date training on chronic pain that's based on current evidence-based ideas, that they stop invalidating and stigmatising patients, that healthcare professionals have the right training to use psychological tools competently, and that there is wider training all-round on gender equity and antiracism.

Another issue faced by people suffering from chronic pain is stigmatising language, which is discussed in that same article. 'The repertoire of terms used to blame clients/patients with pain is extensive. Terms identified in one study of stigmatizing language in hospital admission notes included: difficult patient, drug seeking, fake, in denial, lifestyle disease, malingerer, noncompliant, secondary gain, and unmotivated. Since hospital admission notes are read by all staff who will be providing care, the use of stigmatizing language can have a far-reaching negative impact by influencing the impressions and attitudes of other treating professionals.'[5]

The thing I really struggle with about this research is that it needs to be pointed out in the first place. I don't think it's asking too much to have my GP take me seriously when I go to them in pain. But pain just isn't taught in undergraduate healthcare – a survey of pain education estimated that "the identification, assessment and treatment of pain represent

[5] https://www.jpain.org/article/S1526-5900(23)00471-6/fulltext

less than 1% of the university-based teaching for healthcare professionals'.

It gets worse.

Another study looked at pain being taught at medical schools around the world – this review looked at the curriculum content. Keep in mind that pain is one of the main reasons people go to the doctor in the first place, and one of the most common reasons people go to A&E. Over a third of adult appointments with the GP involve a patient with chronic pain. But 'most people presenting with pain will be treated by a medical practitioner who has not trained as a specialist in pain management. At least 40% of the patients with chronic pain treated in routine practice settings receive inadequate pain management. Newly qualified doctors have expressed a lack of preparedness to deliver prompt and effective management of acute and chronic pain. Primary care providers have indicated a lack of training regarding pain management and limited confidence in their ability to provide effective pain treatment.'[6]

Who's to blame?

'Pain medicine was mostly incorporated into medical courses such as anaesthesia or pharmacology, rather than presented as a dedicated pain medicine module. Ninety-six percent of medical schools in the UK and USA, and nearly 80% of medical schools in Europe had no compulsory dedicated teaching in pain medicine. On average, the median

---

[6] https://pmc.ncbi.nlm.nih.gov/articles/PMC6251835/

number of hours of pain content in the entire curriculum was 20 in Canada (2009), 20 in Australia and New Zealand (2018), 13 in the UK (2011), 12 in Europe (2012/2013), and 11 in the USA (2009).'[7]

Thirteen hours on pain training in the UK? Shouldn't it be a bit more equal? As in, shouldn't doctors spend as much time learning how to treat my pain as I spend being in pain? OK, that's maybe a bit unrealistic, but surely we could do a module on pain? Considering how many of us suffer from it.

In good news, Professor Smith tells me about an important conceptual breakthrough in recent years. 'The International Association for the Study of Pain has now got the World Health Organization to accept the formal diagnosis of what's called chronic primary pain, which is pain for which there is no apparent underlying cause,' Professor Smith says.

This classification recognises chronic pain as a distinct condition, not just a symptom of another disease, and further categorises it into subtypes, including chronic primary pain (MG30.0), chronic cancer-related pain (MG30.1), and chronic post-surgical or post-traumatic pain (MG30.2). The hope here is that this classification will help doctors to diagnose chronic pain with greater accuracy and better manage chronic pain. The upshot? As patients, we'll get better care, and there will be more – and better – research looking into this condition.

What this means is that chronic pain – to doctors and other healthcare providers – is the same in the UK as it is

---

[7] https://pmc.ncbi.nlm.nih.gov/articles/PMC6251835/

in Canada, America, France, Senegal, India, Tahiti. That uniformity helps us to develop and look at disease statistics around the world.

The ICD – the International Classification of Diseases – also captures the things that influence health, which gives us a holistic look at everything – like chronic pain – that affects our health.

Why does any of this matter to you? Because these health statistics form the basis for almost every decision made in healthcare: from understanding what people get sick from, to what eventually kills them, mapping disease trends and epidemics, deciding how to programme health services, allocate healthcare spending, and invest in research and development. All of it is based on statistical evidence. So if chronic pain is included, then it gets counted, and if it gets counted then it matters and it influences important decisions.

ICD codes can have enormous financial importance because they're used to determine where to invest increasingly scant resources. So if chronic pain doesn't show up as itself in these statistics – if it's counted in other places instead – then it doesn't appear important enough to spend money on, to do things like create more pain clinics, or get psychologists into those pain clinics.

The big deal about the ICD is that it gives doctors around the world a shared vocabulary – not only for diagnosing but also for recording, reporting and monitoring health problems. Fifty years ago, it would be unlikely that a disease such as schizophrenia would be diagnosed similarly in Japan, Kenya and Brazil. Now, though, if you see a doctor in Brazil and they can't read your medical records, at least they'll know what the ICD code means.

Most chronic pain is caused by a complex interaction of biological, psychological and social factors. This includes things like chronic widespread pain, fibromyalgia, complex regional pain syndrome type 1 and IBD, along with the usual suspects of back and neck pain conditions. The new classification of chronic primary pain is meant to get rid of the idea that pain is either physical or psychological.

The other useful thing about this kind of standardised classification system is that it lets people figure out the global picture of disease. Part of that picture includes this fact: back and neck pain come in sixth in the top ten global causes of disability-adjusted life years (DALY) in 2021.

If we – as a society – accept that chronic pain is a disease or a long-term condition in its own right, instead of a symptom, then we can treat it that way.

In 1977, George Engel first came up with the idea of something called the biopsychosocial model of pain, which suggested that if you were going to understand someone's medical condition, you had to look at things beyond the biological – you had to include the psychological and social factors.

Mostly what this model means is that your health isn't just down to your doctor. My doctor – my rheumatologist, specifically – is Professor Raj Sengupta, at the Royal National Hospital for Rheumatic Diseases in Bath. This place has a long history of excellence in the management of axial spondyloarthritis (of which ankylosing spondylitis is a specific form) – they're internationally renowned for being at the forefront of care and research into this condition.

When we were talking as part of my research for this book, I said to him that he's the only doctor I've seen in the last twenty or so years who's asked me directly how things are at home, and I asked him why he thought that was.

'Because people don't,' he said. 'This is something I want bring to rheumatology – it's called prehabilitation. When people start on biologics you get variable responses and I think that's because you're only dealing with the inflammatory part of the symptoms. The concept of prehabilitation is helping the person – from a biopsychosocial point of view – to optimise everything they can before they start the biologic. It's about making them as fit and as well as they can be before they start the biologic.'

So often, doctors are all about cytokines and drugs and symptoms. And partly this is because you get fifteen minutes with your doctor in clinic if you're lucky, and this biopsychosocial model takes time.

'Imagine if we said right at start you'll complete these questionnaires. And, in a month, based on those results, you'll go off and do a cognitive behavioural therapy (CBT) programme. In another month, you'll do another module of activities – our goal would be to work out what is the best way to understand the dynamics of the biopsychosocial bit on individual patients.'

Can you imagine a healthcare system where you could go on a full course? I can't. Or even having the time to do this in your life? Me neither. But that doesn't mean it's not a good idea. Professor Sengupta isn't unaware of these challenges and says that the compromise might be to develop digital solutions.

My worry, though, is that digital solutions won't deliver the kind of personal, nuanced care that I'm lucky to receive from the team in Bath.

'I couldn't agree with you more. You've hit the nail on the head. But it's really made me think that this word empathy is so important. But the problem is that if there are a lack of financial resources that would enable us to do the empathy bit, then do we say maybe we shouldn't compromise? Or do we compromise and say we'll try and get as close as we can, even though we don't achieve every bit of what we want to?'

This biopsychosocial approach is really useful too when we're dealing with that newly defined type of pain, nociplastic pain. More and more research is coming out showing that about 25 to 30 per cent of patients with axial spondyloarthritis have fibromyalgia, as well as chronic pain, but as Professor Sengupta says, 'We don't assess this type of pain well enough in the clinic. We don't look for it. Or assess it well enough before someone's starting a biologic.'

Biologics (which are used to treat arthritis, Crohn's and MS, among other conditions) are predominantly dealing with inflammatory pain and not nocioplastic pain. So the patient goes on a biologic, and the score doesn't improve that much, so they try another biologic. 'And nothing's helping the patient because actually, if you fully assessed the patient, you would know that the patient's pain is nociplastic. That they've got chronic pain and you're using the wrong drug to treat it,' Professor Sengupta says.

What that means is that our pain hasn't been properly assessed. You can't be treated for something you don't officially have – as anyone who is undiagnosed but in pain will tell you. What can we do about it? At the rheumatology clinic in Bath, they're now going through the big process of trying to build in questionnaires, and educate doctors, nurses, physiotherapists, to talk about chronic pain and re-assess patients for chronic pain. 'It should be an integral component, which was hit and miss before, but it's so important,' Professor Sengupta says.

Properly assessing pain is sort of where Professor Smith got his start as a researcher. He began with a very simple question. He'd just started his first academic post and a colleague, a pain specialist, wanted to know what percentage of the population has chronic pain so he could make the case for additional resources to the pain service at his hospital. After looking at the literature, he found that there was no good study determining the prevalence of chronic pain. 'And that's partly because there was no accepted definition of what chronic pain was, or if there was a definition, there was no accepted way of identifying people in the community that had it,' he says. 'So we did a bit of research trying to define these things. We devised a questionnaire that defined and identified people with chronic pain in a community-based survey.' Having done that, they organised a much larger community-based survey and found that prevalences of chronic pain were much larger than they'd expected.

'Five per cent of all people and approximately ten per cent of people with chronic pain had the most severe forms. But we also looked at the fact that more women than men had chronic pain and found that prevalence increased with age. It was greater in more deprived areas. It was greater in people who were less educationally qualified, and greater in people with other illnesses and diseases. That all seems well established now, but at the time we were among the first to publish this research,' Professor Smith says. 'We can't do anything about your age and we can't do anything about your biological sex. But knowing that it's more common in more deprived areas means that we need political solutions as well as clinical and drug solutions for preventing it and managing it.'

I mention something called longitudinal studies, which are research studies that follow people for years and years, taking their data so researchers like Professor Smith can look at it to get a bigger picture. He's been involved in those kinds of studies, and also those that look at genetic traits across years, and they've found that there are genetic associations with pain, particularly neuropathic pain. That allows researchers to explore and ask questions around the biology that's associated with these genes and that informs new drugs that might be developed to address those targets. That's the ultimate prize, at least.

There has been some research that drug companies have taken on board and are trying to develop, but the question is how close are we? That's a big unknown in part because so many of the nerve-related mechanisms at play are related to nerve transmission, and a lot of this is to do with the immune system, as we've seen.

Professor Smith goes on to elaborate, echoing a lot of the things other researchers have been saying: 'The problem with pain – as we've discovered in our research – is that it's very, very complex. And the biological factors that underpin pain are only one part of a much more complex picture. The psychology of where you live, who you live with, what your job is, what your previous experiences, what your expectations of treatment are – all these things and many, many more affect the experience of pain. And if we just then block an ion channel, it may not actually have a great effect on the bigger picture. Pain is a multifactorial thing and that understanding probably helps us to address pain as a bigger, more holistic entity. That's certainly where my bias leans, not towards a specific individual molecular solution to pain but the more holistic person-wide, society-wide approach.'

I mention that another researcher illustrated this point by saying that he could give a patient all the biologics in the world, but if that patient was homeless, the biologics weren't going to do much. Pain, in some ways, is a political problem.

'We've worked as closely as we can with Scottish Government,' Professor Smith says. 'I used to be the Scottish Government lead clinician for chronic pain and though I'm no longer involved in that, my successors continue to work with politicians in government to try and seek the kind of approaches that will address these political-medical problems. The medical professionals say it needs political solutions. The politicians say that doctors need to be better and we need better drugs.' If we need a political solution, what are we going to do? Only half-jokingly, I suggest that I might go and see my local MP with my pain and ask them for a political prescription.

Professor Sir Michael Marmot and his team at UCL were asked by the Secretary of State for Health in 2008 to chair an independent review to propose the most effective evidence-based strategies for reducing health inequalities in England. It's called the Marmot Review, and after it was published in 2010, it fundamentally shifted the way we look at and think about health inequalities. As part of the review, Professor Marmot highlighted the importance of giving every child the best start in life. This chimes with what many researchers have said about the importance of adverse childhood events when investigating chronic pain.

Professor Smith has been working a lot recently on identifying the associations between adverse childhood experiences and subsequent chronic pain, drawing similar conclusions to those of Professor Noel. He's particularly interested in how and why women are more likely to experience chronic pain.

First, he feels that women are more likely to experience chronic pain because we live longer, and we know that chronic pain is associated with age. But even within age groups, a lot of the underlying causes of chronic pain are specifically female, such as endometriosis, vulvodynia. And, we know there are genes that are associated with pain in women that are not associated with pain in men.

Fine. But the really interesting part of what he says is this: Sociologically speaking, women are better at attending health services and acknowledging so-called 'weaknesses' than men are. 'Men perhaps express their experiences in different ways. Certainly in the pain clinic, a lot of the people we meet have a lot of really difficult things going on in their lives, and they're expressing that as chronic pain. They're identifying as a person with chronic pain and therefore they come to the pain service.' This is so interesting to me as an idea, that some version of the stereotypical macho male ideal is preventing people from getting help. It's interesting and heartbreaking.

The Centers for Disease Control in the United States did a study that showed women are 33 per cent more likely to visit the doctor than men, and women are 100 per cent better at maintaining screening and preventive care. Nuffield Health says that '65% of men say they avoid seeking medical help for as long as possible when they're unwell, 37% of men say they withhold information from their doctor, and a further 20% admit they aren't always honest during these conversations'.[8] And 41 per cent of men recall being told that 'men don't complain about health issues' as children. Gender stereotypes like this, which get reinforced over time, can contribute to alarming differences in the ways men and women deal with health and wellbeing issues.

Professor Smith tells me that there are instances where people are in chronic pain, but there's no definitive diagnosis. 'There is no doubt that these people have pain, but it's possibly their way of expressing a life of distress. And men,

[8] https://www.nuffieldhealth.com/article/5-reasons-men-avoid-going-to-the-doctor

perhaps, express their distress in ways other than identifying as chronic pain patients, and possibly less healthy ways,' he says. 'Illness is a way that distress can be expressed, and this is absolutely not to say that pain is in anyone's head. The pain is very real. These are genuine symptoms and genuine illnesses, but this is another example of the mind and body working together. I think it's very much the case, particularly in pain, you just can't separate mind and body. Unless you treat one, you won't treat the other.'

Part of why I was particularly interested to talk to Professor Smith is that he's a cancer survivor. I wanted to learn about what chronic cancer pain is like – because it used to be one of the main forms of chronic pain, 'and that was because in treating cancer pain, you basically upped and upped the morphine', because people weren't expected to survive. 'I'm actually lucky to have cancer-related pain because I've survived my cancer and it's eight years since the last cancer was in my body,' he says. In good news, the phrase cancer-survivorship is increasing and people are living longer.

Cancer pain can be caused by the cancer itself and its local effects, and it can be caused when the cancer spreads. Treatment of the cancer using chemotherapy causes 'really nasty neuropathic pain', he says. So does surgery and radiotherapy. 'I think it's slightly artificial to call it cancer pain now unless it's directly related to the tumour I had, which was lots of quite serious surgery for bowel and liver cancer, and as a result of which I've got post-surgical neuropathic pain in my leg, a complication of the of the surgery,' he says. 'That's just there now, and it is what it is.' But it's better than the alternative, which is not having the pain because he's not here.

'I suppose what is important is the attribution of the pain. So you've been able to attribute yours to ankylosing spondylitis, which I know is a really painful and difficult condition. I don't know how you respond to that. With my cancer pain, for example two or three times I've had a recurrence of abdominal pain which has turned out to be just a complication of surgery. But because I've had the history of cancer, and I've got this pain, until I'm certain that it's nothing, I'm wondering if it's the cancer coming back, which makes the pain seem worse and more frightening, and therefore exaggerates it. Then it settles quickly once the diagnosis has been made.' That's an illustration of how the expectations and the associations and the potential causes of pain affect the severity and intensity and impact of the pain. 'Whereas I know this pain I've got in my leg is because the nerve was damaged during the surgery. That's fine. That's what it is. It's not going to get better, but it's not anything to be worried about either. It's just unpleasant,' he says.

I try to think of how that relates to my conditions and experience of pain. New pain is always a worry, because there's always a chance that it'll be some kind of new miserable disease – that's what my experience has been. New pain equals crap new disease. But if it's the old, familiar pain of AS or Crohn's, that's fine. I know where I stand with that pain, I know how to treat it and how to cope with it, which is usually exercise.

I've always felt weirdly fortunate with my diseases – I grew up swimming, and I've spent so much time in a pool that it's become a key part of my life – so I'm in the fortunate position of having exercise I like doing, and that I'm confident doing. But I know that not everyone has grown up feeling confident and comfortable with exercise, and how difficult it can be to be told to 'take some exercise' as an adult with a chronic pain condition, and not even know where to start.

Professor Smith tells me that he and his lab have just published some research, where they've looked at the facilitators and barriers to physical activity in people with chronic pain. It identified the key barriers to regular physical activity for those in chronic pain as being: the impact of pain severity, comorbidities, lack of knowledge about the benefits of physical activity, and time constraints.[9]

Look, I don't know about you, but a highly unscientific canvassing of my friends tells me that the barriers to exercise are generally: I don't like it or don't want to do it; I hurt so I can't; I'm too busy; I find gyms unpleasant or too expensive. When I spoke with Professor Sengupta about the exercise point, he said they've been wracking their brains for ages trying to figure out how to motivate people to exercise, and they've come up with nothing. My experience tells me that you need to start young and you need to be able to see the benefits.

'I think physical activity is better, and more likely to lead to success than the drug discovery research arising from the genetic studies,' Professor Smith says. More important than

---

[9] https://journals.lww.com/pain/pages/articleviewer.aspx?year=2024&issue=12000&article=00010&type=Fulltext

drug discovery? What does he think will be the next big breakthrough, then, in chronic pain? 'I think it's going to be a shared understanding by health services and the population that management of chronic pain is not based on drugs.

'It is hard for people to accept and some people won't accept it. Take, for example, opioids. That's morphine and codeine, and these drugs – a lot of people that we see in the pain service have been on opioids for years and years and years and it's going to be very difficult to get them off it. But starting at the other end, I think we're now much more at the stage where there's a much greater reluctance to start people on opioids, so they don't get to the stage of long-term opioid use, and if they do start them, then it's for very short term with very clear goals to be achieved and with an exit plan at the end.'

Now, I know there are people with my disease (and, of course, others) who are on opioid-based medications, and I've seen them write about how difficult it is to keep getting their scripts. And how sometimes they're flat-out refused. When I mention that to Professor Smith, he says, 'The worst thing is to suddenly stop opioids both because of withdrawal effects, but also because of the lack of support that it implies. It is cruel and it's an extreme response that we would certainly never promote. I would certainly never, nor would my colleagues in the pain service, ever promote abruptly stopping that for people who are already on those drugs. We would bring them in, and have discussions about the long-term effects of being an opioid.' Based on evidence of the ineffectiveness of opioids long term, and their harms, the medical profession is much more reluctant to start people on opioids.

But for us patients, Professor Smith believes that the next important thing we need to do is to change patient expectations around morphine. How are we going to do that? 'I think that's public education. I think more people are aware of the opioid crisis. I think people, especially people who are lucky to receive more education – and this comes back to health inequalities – are more reluctant to take opioids,' he says. This, for me, is part of the work that I think we need to do in getting the latest research into clinics. At my day job, I spend a lot of time talking about translational medicine, about turning research into new treatments – mostly drugs.

But it also seems to me that, actually, we need to change the transactional way we approach doctors and prescriptions and pain. This idea reminds me of something my old rheumatologist in Toronto, Dr Keystone, used to tell me. He'd always talk about working *with* me, as a patient. Which gave me a sense of shared responsibility. Now, I know that people in chronic pain do a lot as far as daily coping and taking care of ourselves, and that sometimes just getting out of bed is as much as we can do on a given day. I don't want to or intend to cast any of us in a light that might imply we're shirking our duties, or that we should do more heavy lifting and our doctors should do less. Rather, what I think might be the most useful is if we all look at it like a partnership, and that everyone needs to put a bit more time in, but that everyone should also get more support to do that.

But we need resources and training to provide that multidisciplinary support. There's of course peer to peer support – things like Facebook groups, WhatsApp chats – and

Professor Smith tells me about a pain toolkit, which I hadn't come across before. It was set up by a guy named Pete Moore who has back pain and decided he didn't want to be on opioids. So he found his own way. It's all about self-management. He tries to put people like us in the driving seat. And it's a great resource, but it's vulnerable to the vagaries of third-sector funding and the ongoing energy of the individuals who run it. Mostly, it feels like the way forward here is the mutual understanding and the expectation that managing chronic pain isn't done by just taking a pill.

Another researcher who tells me that treating chronic pain is about more than taking tablets is Stefan Siebert, Professor of Inflammation Medicine and Rheumatology. His bio on the University of Glasgow's website says: 'As clinical researcher, he is involved in managing patients with rheumatoid and other types of inflammatory arthritis, studying mechanisms that underlie these conditions and running clinical trials of new therapies.

His research is focused on psoriatic arthritis and spondyloarthritis, and in comparing how the underlying immune processes differ from rheumatoid arthritis. This approach has the potential to yield information about the specific underlying mechanisms and possible therapeutic targets for each of these conditions. He is also interested in understanding the effects of current arthritis therapies using a variety of immunological, laboratory and health informatics approaches.'[10]

---

[10] https://www.gla.ac.uk/schools/infectionimmunity/staff/stefansi ebert/#biography

What that means in practice is that his research group does a bit of epidemiology, things like using UK Biobank to understand population level stuff that's going on in those diseases, and he also does a bit of work on rheumatoid arthritis, 'because it's a generalised inflammatory arthritis so serves as a good comparator'. A lot of the work they do is around trying to understand how drugs work. 'Because even though they're targeted, we don't always know exactly how they work or why they do in some people and not in others. We're also trying to see if we can find biomarkers to predict who's going to respond, who's going to develop problems. At the moment, prescribing these drugs is still largely trial and error,' he says.

For the drugs, their interest is in stratifying patients. For example, with targeted therapies, can they understand who will benefit and who won't before giving them to the patient? To figure that out they look at biomarkers and tissue biopsies for psoriatic arthritis. Often, Professor Siebert says, they also use the drugs as a way to better understand inflammation and the diseases themselves.

As part of a larger group, he and his colleagues do brain imaging to understand the fatigue that's part of these chronic diseases. 'Fatigue is still poorly understood, and it's certainly not improved to the same level by these drugs,' Professor Siebert says. They also work with an immunology neuropsychiatrist, who is interested in what happens with depression and mood in the brain in response to inflammation. 'We tend to do everything from basic science, immunology through clinical work through to a bit of epidemiology, population level,' he says.

I cut right to the chase and ask about the potential for CAR T-cell therapy. 'I think CAR T is harder for these diseases. Partly because you have to know what the cell is that you're targeting – targeting specific T cells or the B cells makes a lot of sense in lupus. It's a brilliant model for it. However, we still need to understand the problem cells in these diseases and what we know about AS, for example, is that the blood immune signature can be pretty bland,' he says. I've never heard blood described as bland before. 'What I mean by that is it's not like rheumatoid arthritis, where there's a lot of inflammation going on and detectable in blood. AS is much more subtle and a lot of it probably happens at the tissue level in the spine. There are relatively few cells circulating in blood that are actually the culprits or detectable. There isn't a whole group of cells you could easily target. There's a very small number of those, but I think our technologies are getting better to start finding them. And once we find them instead of trying to suppress everything, we can really get much more targeted.'

But that's probably pretty far off for my disease. For things like psoriatic arthritis and Crohn's, he thinks it's a bit closer. But he cautions me, because 'it's expensive at the moment and risky – let's not get away from that'. And he's right – it's all fine and well to want new treatments and the possibility of a cure, but if only wealthy people like us who live in the richest countries can afford them, that's not equitable. I suppose another way of framing that question is that we're not really treating the disease if we spend valuable time and research funding on developing treatments only for the wealthy. In that case, we're just treating ourselves.

For drugs that target diseases where we haven't got great treatments it's going to be more of an issue. With AS, drugs like methotrexate were tried and didn't work, then researchers moved on to the targeted biologics, which block a single biologic pathway. 'We borrowed ideas from rheumatoid arthritis and then we learned from psoriasis and psoriatic arthritis and Crohn's, and that's where we got to interleukin inhibitors and then we moved on to the JAK inhibitors, which can block a number of pathways. I think we still don't know exactly which JAK is the best for which disease, but we're getting better,' he says. JAKs and interleukins are part of signalling pathways involved in inflammatory and immune responses.

There are some new JAK inhibitors coming out, and they'll probably have better safety and hopefully as good efficacy. 'In terms of the next line of drugs that are coming, these are aiming to address one of the worries with the big antibodies (biologic cytokine and interleukin blockers) that they don't get into the target tissue itself,' he says. TNF-inhibitors get in the blood – so they're brilliant for rheumatoid arthritis where there is lots of inflammation in the blood, and also quite good for many other inflammatory diseases, but they don't get into your tissues as they are too large. Now researchers are looking if small nanobodies can deliver the treatments directly to the tissues. Can it really get in the tissue? We need to see if that's needed or if that's going to lead to a big change for patients, because maybe just inhibiting the antibodies a little bit in the blood is enough. That's what pharma is really interested in now: how to get the same drugs into the tissues, including the spine joints in AS.

'Rheumatoid arthritis is a disease that is active in the blood and then affects the joints, so it made sense that treating the inflammation in the blood made rheumatoid arthritis better. I think we got a bit lucky with psoriatic arthritis and AS – that TNF inhibitors worked so well for these says there is enough going on in the blood that can be targeted. One reason we don't get as good results (in psoriatic arthritis) may be because that's not enough, perhaps we need medicines that get into the tissues as well,' Professor Siebert says. The antibodies are huge relative to other molecules and these much smaller nanobodies will, due to their size and chemistry, potentially get into the tissues, and maybe that's better because there aren't many drugs that go to the spine. And to the brain even less, although we still don't know if that will be a good or bad thing, or perhaps both.

I ask what his motivation was to focus on inflammation and pain. It was a very personal story. He grew up South Africa, and it was 'all trauma and HIV'. In the UK, he was better able to focus on medicine and rheumatology in particular. What he liked about rheumatology was that it was whole-body and whole-person medicine – for example, a cardiologist just listens to the heart. 'They don't ever look if a person's got a rash or other issues and it just bugs me. I like whole-body medicine and inflammation is whole-body medicine,' he says.

'It is worth remembering that rheumatology was essentially a rehab specialty in the past – we used to have wards full of people with rheumatoid arthritis, and we couldn't treat them well. All we could do was give them physio, steroids and pain killers, and it was depressing.' The biologic drugs were a game-changer. With something like rheumatoid arthritis, doctors can get 'the fire under control with drugs', and it's probably a bit easier than with something like AS. 'Rheumatoid is mainly just the fire (inflammation), and as a clinician, you can be more confident when pain isn't due to ongoing inflammation. So, in other words, you can manage pain as pain. The problem we have in AS is that it's so hard to see the spine – even when with specialist imaging. Is your back pain because you've still got ongoing inflammation and you need a new biologic, or is it because of some other reason or structural things?' he says. 'The inflammation can be at such a low level you're never quite sure – am I missing inflammation? Do I need to focus on treating the pain?' The problem is working out what is causing the pain and how best to treat this.

The one thing doctors and researchers can't do with our pain is treat the socioeconomic problems driving some of this. Professor Siebert does his clinics in the East End of Glasgow, an area that has high levels of deprivation. 'This is just anecdotal, but there are some patients who have always attended clinic regularly but then they stop coming. When I phone them to follow up, what you find is some of them have been made homeless and so they haven't received their biologic (you need an address for this to be delivered to), or they haven't got a fridge to store this medication – prescribing more medicine is not going to solve that. It's just shocking. How can we treat their arthritis, let alone get their pain under control? All you can try to do is be supportive and see what you can do to help.' But even that support system is struggling. 'In the old days we used to do letters to the social services and something happened, but now often nothing happens,' he says.

'I can usually make people's disease better but I can't make their lives better. I think we shouldn't underestimate the effects these things have on people's pain. I've got people using food banks and it's totally demoralising, because you want to help people. The way some doctors cope, unfortunately, with patients in that scenario is they stop caring. They think, Well, I've treated your inflammation so off you go as there's nothing more I can do, which is terrible. Or they keep trying to use more drugs to treat inflammation that isn't there, but they still don't make things better. And so it's hard. I think a lot of doctors just don't want to think about it sometimes because it's not our thing – we make people better. And if you can't, you're a failure. Some doctors don't ask about your pain or your life. I've got some patients whose lives are so hard – you wouldn't believe what they go through and I sometimes can't believe it. The solution is not for me to give them another drug because that'll make me feel better, but it won't make them better and puts them at other risks. I try to help them with the other things.' It's getting worse, too, with the increase in the cost of living. 'That's why I don't think we'll ever get rid of everyone's pain, just like we won't get everyone out of poverty. But I think we can do a hell of a lot better.

'We also don't have psychologists to support our patients. We have made business cases for psychologists without success, and for pain relief even just getting seen in a pain clinic, people often have to wait for ages. And when some people do get seen in a pain clinic, the team say, "Oh, you've got rheumatoid arthritis or AS. See your rheumatologist." It's just passing the buck back – there's a structural service problem here,' he adds.

'The other thing that's not said is obviously pain isn't visible, not only for employers but also for the government. There has to be more than just saying as long as people are working, things are OK. People are in pain. It's not cancer, so it's underfunded. But I would argue that if you could "solve pain", then you'd boost the economy much more than you would with anything else because people would be able to be more productive and do their work better, especially with regards to musculoskeletal pain. It would be a game changer, for these patients' quality of life and for society in general.'

HOW TO IMPROVE CHRONIC PAIN RESEARCH 11

Despite having heard a lot about all the other ways we can mitigate chronic pain, I can't help thinking about drugs. They've still got the potential to help, but the longer I think about that, the more I start to wonder where all the new drugs are. When I speak to Professor Jeffrey Mogil, E. P. Taylor Chair in Pain Studies at McGill University in Montreal, part of the answer becomes clearer. There are, from his point of view, a few things the research community could be doing better. He singles out animal models as being a big problem, the measures in our assays (by which he means how we put animals in pain), and the subjects we use in experiments as places where, to put it gently, improvements could be made.

'I think the problem is that the animal models have been instantiated in the wrong ways so that they're not relevant to the clinical problem,' he says. He thinks that 'they're measuring something, just not the thing we want them to measure'. The problem with the subjects researchers use is that there is an entire universe of genotypes – genetic backgrounds – to do pain research on. We can't do it on humans for obvious reasons, so we have to use animals, and for rather arbitrary reasons, we decided that 'not only are we gonna do all the research on mice and rats, we're going to stick with young adult male rats, specifically Sprague Dawley ones. For mice, it's a similar situation: young male adults, specifically the C57BL/ 6 variety.'

As Professor Mogil puts it: 'The problem, especially in mice, is not only do we primarily use one strain, it's an inbred strain, which is a just a terrible idea. And we've done that because it's convenient.'

This is, for Professor Mogil, one of the biggest problems: 'No one is incentivising me to cure pain. What I am being incentivised directly to do is to publish as many papers as possible in the highest impact journals possible. That's what I'm incentivised to do. And because I'm incentivised to do that, I need to collect the most data possible, because that's what reviewers want. They want to be bowled over with data, and the way to bowl them over with data with finite funding is to do the cheapest, fastest experiments possible that will pass muster.'

Researchers, he says, use inbred mice because they think they'll be able to use fewer of them, and that will make experiments cheaper. Rodent models are used in the first place because 'they're the cheapest mammals that we can keep alive'. And with mice, a lot of them can be kept in a room together. Reducing costs like this helps generate as much sample size as possible per unit of time and dollar. 'That's the problem with subjects: we've limited ourselves to this unrepresentative, tiny little subpopulation of a couple species,' he says.

The next problem, as he sees it, is around the assays that researchers are using. For clinical pain that involves inflammation, researchers are going to need a body part that's inflamed, and in mouse or rat models that's almost always the hind paw because it's the easiest to get to. Researchers inject a solution that causes inflammation and we say that's kind of like arthritis, because arthritis is an inflammatory disease. Another example is nerve damage – a lot of pain is caused because of nerve damage, so to better understand that, researchers damage some nerves in an animal's hind paw. 'And that's going to be kind of like – or close enough – to post-herpetic neuralgia or diabetic neuropathy,' he says. I can tell by the look on his face how much he's baffled by the choices we're making.

As I'm listening to Professor Mogil talk it seems so obvious what's wrong with the system. The way we're measuring pain doesn't take into account all the other things that are almost certainly contributing to pain. 'It's true that most pain is inflammation or nerve damage, so that if you create inflammation or nerve damage, you are kind of modelling it. But not really,' he says. We're sort of mimicking our human experiences of pain in these rodent models. And yes, they're models so they're not meant to be exact, that's why we have human clinical trials, but the point that Professor Mogil is at pains to make is that if we did better with these models, then maybe we'd get better answers.

The question is, then, could we do better? Professor Mogil smiles and leans forward. 'I'm going to tell you a story,' he says. In 2012 or thereabouts he had a grad student, Melissa Farmer, and she developed a mouse model of vulvodynia – which is pain, burning and/or discomfort in the vulva. It might affect up to 12 per cent of childbearing-age women, and it's the most common pain disorder that no one's ever heard of. So they developed an animal model for the disorder. At the time, there was this idea in the clinical community that patients who were treated for vulvodynia had more than their fair share of yeast infections. Professor Mogil and (now) Dr Farmer wondered if vulvodynia was something secondary to recurrent yeast infections. They gave mice yeast infections and then treated the yeast infections with fluconazole, and waited for it to clear up. Then they gave the mice another yeast infection and cleared that up, and so on and so forth. After three or four or five rounds, the mice started developing permanent vulva pain – the exact symptom of vulvodynia. They also had other histochemical changes that looked exactly like what is reported in people with vulvodynia.

Professor Mogil was sharing the findings and saying this was not an animal *model* – they'd actually given mice vulvodynia. It was identical to vulvodynia in humans. And how many times did anyone else in the world ever use that assay – that method of giving the mice the same disease via infection over and over again? Zero. Why? Because of the time it took to create the disease. Researchers just don't have that kind of time to work in this way.

Arguably, measuring is even more of an obvious problem. 'The scientific community doesn't agree on a way to measure spontaneous pain yet,' Professor Mogil says. Why should you care? If we're measuring something that's different to what we're experiencing, then we're never going to get drugs to treat our pain.

The number one symptom of human chronic pain is spontaneous pain. What does that mean? Say your arm hurts. The pain is coming from inside the arm and it's there at rest and it's there if nothing's touching it. That's the number one symptom of chronic pain. There are other symptoms like tenderness to touch (called mechanical allodynia), abnormal pain responses to heat or cold stimuli (called thermal hyperalgesia). These are less prevalent and less bothersome than spontaneous pain, and so you would imagine that the number one priority would be to measure spontaneous pain in mice and rats. Do we do that? No, we do not.

Professor Mogil says that researchers think the assays that they're using to give rodents pain are giving mice and rats spontaneous pain, but is that really what's being measured? His view is that they're mostly measuring mechanical and thermal hypersensitivity. Why? Because it's easy. 'You poke them with something, or use heat beams or cold stimuli, and they withdraw. And you say, Ah, look, pain. But it's not the same pain people present in clinic with, it's mechanical or thermal hypersensitivity, which turns out to be completely different symptoms with completely different biologies than spontaneous pain,' he says. 'We're ignoring the number one symptom because we don't know how to measure it, and we can't agree on how to measure it, and all the ways to measure it are more complex.'

Is there a way to measure spontaneous pain? Yes, and it has got better recently and includes things like facial expressions of pain, which Professor Mogil's lab developed. And in rodent models, researchers can also measure place preference to analgesics, and changes in normal behaviours like digging and burrowing. 'There are lots of different things that have been suggested, but they're all much more work than poking,' he says.

Another key challenge is that researchers are ignoring all kinds of laboratory environmental factors that are affecting experiments. For example, more than one mouse in the cage can mess up results. Why? They can affect each other's pain behaviours. Professor Mogil's lab showed in 2014 that human experimenters can affect mouse pain behaviour, if they're men, by causing something called olfactory-mediated analgesia.

Professor Mogil's team measured the response from mice and rats to an injection given in the ankle, either with different experimenters in the room, or after the people had left and the rodents were alone. The animals seemed to show a decrease in pain response of about 40 per cent when a man stayed in the room. A T-shirt that a man had worn the night before and put in the room with the animals had the same effect, as did the smell of certain chemicals from the armpit that are at higher levels in men than women. A woman's presence – either in person, or from the smell of a T-shirt – didn't alter the pain response at all, and researchers noticed that in fact it seemed to counteract the response to men.[1]

---

[1] https://www.nature.com/articles/nature.2014.15106#:~:text=Rats and mice show increased,animal studies, the study suggests.

So what's the deal with that? Mogil's team dug a little deeper and discovered that the men stressed the animals out, and that stress temporarily quashed the rodent pain response. And the thing here is that this skews results, which makes it harder to develop new drugs: if your mouse models are showing a reduction in pain, you want to know for sure that it's your drug that's doing it, not some smelly man's armpit.

What Professor Mogil tells me next blows my mind: it turns out that the more you test for pain, the longer that pain lasts. 'We have assays that we think we produce pain for a month, but actually they only produce pain for something like four days. Why do we see that? It lasts for a month because we keep testing the mice. If you just leave the mice on the shelf and then take them out a month later, you find that where there would normally be pain you don't see anything.'

The reason the pain seems to last so long is that researchers keep taking them off the shelf, putting them into the same room and poking them over and over again to measure their pain. They've been in that room before, and the last time they were in that room a bad thing happened. The mice aren't stupid; they've been conditioned. They've learned. I suppose it's just like how our brains learn a pain response when, say, we're going up stairs.

Finally, what about duration? Chronic pain in humans lasts three months or more, which is arbitrary, sure, but the average amount of time in 2024 that a mouse pain experiment lasts is two weeks. Researchers take their baseline measurements, give them an injury, test after the injury, and then two weeks later the experiment is done. 'We've developed this idea that because mice and rats only live for two or three years, that three months in 'mouse time' is three days. But is that how chronic pain develops? Those events involved in the transition from acute to chronic pain aren't happening faster in mice – if they were, we'd know. The mouse nerves don't conduct faster; the molecular events happening inside the mouse are unfolding at the same speed as our own. The point is that maybe three months in mouse time is actually just three months. And, if that's the case, and there are only a couple of dozen studies that have ever looked at chronic pain in mice and rats, then it's no wonder things are failing to translate. We're developing drugs that work against acute mechanical allodynia and we're surprised when those drugs don't work against chronic pain in humans, which is spontaneous and has been around for four years.' Of course it doesn't work; it was developed for a completely different situation.

He adds quickly, that 'there are a lot of people who believe that the problem is that the clinical trials have been compromised'. Which sounds shocking. 'And one of the ways that the clinical trials have been compromised is – and we've published a paper about this – is that the response in the placebo arm of the trial has been going up over time such that it's harder and harder to beat placebo. And to the extent that that's true, if we do come up with something that really works, we may never be able to prove it until we can fix what's going wrong with the clinical trials.'

Placebo arms are when you take part in a drug trial and they give some people the new drug, and some people get a pill that's nothing, a placebo. They're how scientists can tell if their drug is making a difference. The paper his research group published in 2014 showed that the people in the placebo arm of neuropathic pain trials get on average 30 per cent better during the trial from placebo. So if a drug is going to beat placebos, it has to do better than 30 per cent, and that's hard to do. And since fewer and fewer drugs do that, fewer and fewer get approved.

Professor Mogil tells me about something called 'numbers-needed-to-treat' (NNT), which is a formula that helps understand how well drugs work. For example, if your NNT is four, what that means is that you need to treat four people with your drug to get just one of them to respond who wouldn't have already responded to placebo. That's the important bit. It doesn't mean only one patient is going to get better; it means that only one patient of the four is going to get better because of your drug.

For neuropathic pain (nerve pain), NNTs start at about four, and then they get worse. 'And again, this is a glass half empty, glass half full question, right? You could take an NNT of five and say that at least it works 20 per cent of the time. That's better than nothing. But I would say that a drug with an NNT of five doesn't work and we should stop pretending that it does. Because when a drug like pregabalin is considered the "gold standard" and has an NNT of six, that's an ineffective drug. All we're saying by calling it a gold standard is that its side effects aren't too bad, but basically it doesn't work,' he says, before adding: 'What I would say is that for chronic pain, nothing works. We don't have anything that works. And it might be better if we all just start admitting that.'

WHAT IF PAIN ISN'T DRIVEN BY THE BRAIN? 12

'The one other major thing I want to tell you about,' says Professor Mogil, 'around where the pain world is going is this: I am increasingly convinced that the following two facts – which appear to contradict each other – are both true. And it's the question about whether pain is all in your head. Now, first thing I should say is that pain is clearly not in anyone's head, in the sense that no one's making it up. The idea that a person not really in pain would go and make multiple appointments with multiple doctors for a thing that didn't exist, that's insane.'

He means 'in our head' in another sense. The two facts? He believes that it's becoming increasingly clear that everyone with chronic pain has had some sort of pathology: 'They either have inflammation that no one can see – we now know that there is this chronic low-level inflammation all over the place that doesn't have the usual markers of inflammation. So it doesn't show up as inflammation, but it's inflammation. It has the same negative effects.'

'Or people have nerve damage that no one can see. And what does that mean? If you have nerve damage to a large fibre, it shows up on a scan. But if you have nerve damage of a very small fibre, the only way to know is to do something called a punch biopsy followed by a very special histology, but there are only three or four labs in the world that do that. And what it would show is that you've lost all your nerve fibres or maybe you have too many nerve fibres. Either way, it's nerve damage,' he says.

Professor David Andersson, at King's College London, is also of the view that pain isn't driven by the brain. How did he arrive at that conclusion? 'We started with cells,' he says. 'The molecules we were very interested in were ion channel proteins, which are thought to be responsible for our ability to touch, understand temperature and so on.' Most of their work was focused on the idea that altered function in those channels could be responsible for pain. 'But we had all of these different experimental models of producing sensitivity in animals, of producing neuropathy-like conditions in mice. I then became increasingly interested in the fact that we don't actually have models that accurately represent anything that is common in the clinic.'

Professor Andersson's research group has been focused on the potential role of antibodies, and much of that work has been focused on complex regional pain syndrome (CRPS). They showed that mice who were given an injury (a small skin incision) and then given antibodies from people who had CPRS didn't recover. Those that received antibodies from control individuals were unchanged, precisely like naive mice.

'So we are firmly of the view that most or perhaps almost all common pain conditions are not in fact driven by the brain as literature may have you believe,' he says.

His team recently made an exciting breakthrough in understanding fibromyalgia: showing that many of the symptoms in fibromyalgia syndrome are caused by antibodies that increase the activity of pain-sensing nerves throughout the body. The results show that fibromyalgia is a disease of the immune system, rather than the currently held view that it originates in the brain. 'We have shown that patient antibodies make several types of nerve fibres that are important for pain hyperactive.'

Their research shows that increased pain sensitivity, muscle weakness, reduced movement and reduced number of small nerve-fibres in the skin – all typical of fibromyalgia – are a consequence of patient antibodies. Professor Andersson's team injected mice with antibodies from people living with fibromyalgia and the mice quickly developed an increased sensitivity to pressure and cold, as well as displaying reduced movement and paw grip strength. In contrast, mice that were injected with antibodies from healthy people were totally fine.

The really exciting bit is that the mice who were injected with fibromyalgia antibodies recovered after a few weeks when the antibodies had been cleared from their system. Which means that therapies aimed at reducing antibody levels in patients are likely to be effective treatments. These kinds of therapies are already available and are used to treat other disorders that are caused by autoantibodies.

How do those therapies work? 'Antibodies are best known for their ability to defend us against infections,' Professor Andersson says. 'We make them against viruses and bacteria and other infections, but we do also all produce some autoantibodies. They are often without any negative consequences or impact, and some of them may in fact have physiological roles. We don't know very much about them, but for example I'm type one diabetic. I have antibodies that destroyed my insulin producing cells. If you have a rheumatic disease, antibodies are most likely involved in some aspects of the disorder.'

In fibromyalgia there aren't inflammatory or destructive processes, and we think of autoimmune conditions as doing precisely that – they inflame and destroy. For example, joint tissue is destroyed when you have antibodies finding and activating immune cells to produce inflammatory and destructive processes. But we know that we can have lifelong presence of antibodies without any destructive inflammatory processes. So Professor Andersson thinks that we have similar mechanisms operating in fibromyalgia – that we have antibodies which change the function of the target instead of activating immune cells to destroy the target cells.

If you've got fibromyalgia, you're probably wondering what they're doing with this knowledge. They want to make a diagnostic test, and to do that they're looking for a target, which would be a lot easier if they knew what the antibodies were likely to bind to. But they don't – yet – so they, and others, are using a lot of approaches to find one.

They're also really excited about what will be found in clinical trials looking for proof of efficacy of drugs or treatments that reduce antibody levels, some of which were developed for myasthenia gravis (an autoimmune disease that causes muscle weakness). If the findings match their thinking, they should work – as a treatment for fibromyalgia – without them knowing the target. 'If we knew the target, we can actually fish out only those antibodies we think are responsible for problems and clear them from patients. It would be an absolute game-changer for people with fibromyalgia,' Professor Andersson says.

He's not the only researcher who has made exciting discoveries around where pain is originating outside of the brain. I read about a new research breakthrough made by Dr Guy Bewick, Associate Professor, University of Aberdeen, and Professor Chih-Cheng, of Academia Sinica in Taiwan. He and Dr Bewick ended up collaborating by accident – a moment of pure serendipity. 'We were both working on different problems, but we found commonality between them,' Dr Bewick says. 'Professor Chen was the one who noticed that my lab group were working on these ion channels. And that's when we started collaborating.

'One of the things I stress whenever I can is the importance of blue skies research. You never know when the bit of information that you uncover will be important. We need to do directed translational research, disease-focused research. But if you're always looking under the light where you know everything and can see it clearly, you won't know what's happening in the dark. Blue skies research is showing light in the dark. And to me that intersection can be very, very powerful.' He's right – if the discovery research or basic foundational science hasn't been done, then there's nothing to translate into a new drug. 'People forget that first step,' Dr Bewick continues. 'They say, "Oh, we've got to fix this disease. We've identified what it is." But if you don't know everything about the system, then you're missing potential clues as to how you might treat that disease. You only know what you know now. You don't know what you don't know. You've got to go and have a look.'

He and Professor Chen have been looking at the peripheral mechanism of pain, and how that leads to chronic pain. The main idea – which we've heard from many of the researchers here – is that there's something that goes wrong in the brain and central nervous system. But, as Professor Chen – who is speaking to me after eleven o'clock at night in Taiwan, so keen is he to discuss the research – says, 'This kind of story doesn't tell you whether the peripheral input continues.' What does he mean by peripheral input? The central nervous system is the brain and spinal cord. They're enclosed and kept within the blood–brain barrier. The peripheral environment is everything else – for example, the nerves that go out from the spinal cord and brain, to and from your muscles and your skin. All of those are the peripheral nervous system. So, we do feel the pain centrally because we're aware of it. We 'know' it's there. But that doesn't mean it's not being caused by something in our peripheral nerves constantly firing off and telling us that the pain is there.

What Dr Bewick and Professor Chen have focused on is fibromyalgia which, in their words, is a 'typical chronic pain'.

In their mouse model of fibromyalgia, they found a surprising interplay between pain nerve endings and muscle spindles. Muscle spindles are special organs inside muscles formed early in development by nerve endings, which capture some of the muscle cells within spring-like structures. Those nerve endings, with their captured muscle fibres, are enclosed in a capsule. This produces a feedback system that tells your body if your muscles, and your limbs, are moving – either by you (because your brain is sending instructions) or something else (like an earthquake).

If you expect to move then you feel that you're in control of your limbs, which is essential for walking without tripping. But if you tell your limbs to move and they don't, you know they're trapped. So, spindles report muscle length all the time. 'It's like having a SatNav. You need to know where you are to start off with to plan a route to your destination – you need to have the initial feedback saying this is where you're starting from in order to get to where you want to be. And that's the same with your limbs,' Dr Bewick says. 'Every muscle in your body – or just about (there's always exceptions in biology) – has these nerve endings which tell you where your limbs are.' This length detection, along with our sense of touch (which monitors skin and joint ligament stretch) is called 'proprioception', the ability to sense the position, movement and action of your body in space without looking.

When muscle is stretched, muscle spindles generate an electrical signal which tells you you've moved. Dr Bewick's research team, along with his collaborator for over 25 years, Dr Robert Banks of Durham University, found that the length-detecting proprioceptive nerve endings inside the spindles also release glutamate. So, when you stretch them, they release a chemical, and that doesn't make any sense at all. They don't need to release that chemical, as they've already felt the stimulus and they've already generated the electrical signal. 'What we noticed was that if you stop the glutamate secretion, then the ending turns off. And if you put glutamate on, then the ending fires more when you stretch it,' Dr Bewick says. 'But we didn't know what the glutamate was for exactly. It could either have been very interesting or all we were doing was in some way over stimulating the nerve by adding glutamate. But we found that the glutamate ending becomes more responsive to its proper stimulus, firing more during the same movement.' Essentially, it becomes more sensitive. When it gets turned on by a stretch, the response is louder, like turning the volume up on a radio.

Around 70 per cent of the synapses in the brain use glutamate to communicate. It's an excitatory transmitter, so it's used very widely by the central nervous system just for sending signals. 'But in the periphery, it's very rare to find it. It's always in the central nervous system for neurons to talk to each other, but in the periphery it's nearly always something else, which is why it was a big surprise to find glutamate in the proprioceptors,' Dr Bewick says. 'Even the proprioceptor nerves, when they get into the central nervous system – they release glutamate from that end to tell the brain that something's happening to your muscles. What we were surprised at is that it's also found at the other end of the nerve, where it's in the muscle. And that's really what's so special about it – its location.'

Having discovered the glutamate secretion system in this muscle nerve fibre capsule system, they reasoned there must be receptors for the glutamate to activate to get the increased sensitivity. And they found something that had never been identified before: a highly unusual glutamate receptor arrangement on the sensory nerve endings for proprioception. 'Eventually we pinned it down to this thing called GluK2,' Dr Bewick says. 'Which is a protein that rarely appears by itself. It usually has lots of friends.' They also found a way to block it, 'and that means the glutamate has no effect anymore'.

Researchers also learned that there are acid-sensing ion channels – ASICs – on proprioceptor (muscle spindle nerve) endings. ASICs act like pores (a hole into the cell), allowing specific ions to pass through. They're really important for a lot of things, not least of which is mediating nerve firing. Professor Chen's research had recently shown some pain nerves also have these ASICs, where they respond to acid build-up in muscles by signalling that it's painful.

Dr Bewick and Professor Chen see it like this: in proprioceptor nerve endings the ASIC channels are the on/off switch of movement detection. If they're there, they're opened by movement, causing an electrical signal that triggers the proprioceptor nerve to fire. This happens very quickly – detecting even the tiniest movement as soon as it happens. What the glutamate does is much longer term – and Dr Bewick's team think it controls the number of ASIC channels present on the nerve ending surface. For 30–60 minutes after a stretch it controls how many ASICs are on the surface, which changes how much firing will be done and how loud the signal should be.

So, the glutamate secretion is triggered by opening ASIC channels on proprioceptor endings in muscle spindles. That's where Professor Chen noticed that there could be crosstalk between the glutamate release from proprioceptors and pain fibres. Humans, like mice, also have ASICs in some pain-sensing fibres, so when you inject the acid it activates both sets of ASICs. 'Perhaps this arrangement is what makes the muscles hypersensitive to pain,' says Professor Chen.

Professor Chen thinks that the pain turns chronic because of repeated over-stimulation of this system. In mice, if you inject acid into a muscle the first time, it induces an increased sensitivity to touch, or sng-pain in Taiwanese, by opening ASIC channels on the pain fibres. This goes away in 24 hours. But if you inject acid again into the same muscle within five days, the mice develop chronic increased sensitivity lasting for more than three weeks – and it can never turn off even when painkillers are applied. The double stimulation has produced chronic pain. 'You need the first trigger – it seems to prime the system to be ready in case there is a second trigger. Essentially, your system is learning,' says Professor Chen.

What they think is happening is that the acid is activating the ASICs on the pain fibres and the ASICs on the muscle spindle terminals, where it produces excessive glutamate release. They think that the acid activates the ASICs in both types of nerve. In the pain fibres, it triggers a little effect the first time, but it contributes to pain chronicity the second time the acid is injected. In the proprioceptors, it triggers excessive glutamate release, and the extra glutamate spills onto the nearby pain fibres. The result is that the nerve thinks – because of this excessive glutamate – that something serious might be happening, so get ready. If it happens again, something seriously damaging is probably happening and it needs to be really super-sensitive from now on. The priming and second trigger need to be close together to get chronic pain. If you wait a long time (more than five days in the mouse model), then everything goes back to normal. But, if these two things happen twice in a short period of time, the pain doesn't turn off.

Part of the work these two teams have done is to then try to reframe this acid-induced chronic muscle pain as something called 'sng'. Professor Chen explains it like this: 'We have different types of chronic pain. So what we're calling sng is another type of chronic pain.' The concept is embedded in Taiwanese culture, and it's different because it's triggered by the proprioceptors. 'It also explains why some types of chronic pain are difficult to treat,' Professor Chen says. 'If we do the double acid injection, the pain comes on and it's chronic. But if we block this glutamate receptor in the proprioceptor, we no longer get chronic pain.'

They are keen to stress that this does not show how to turn off chronic pain; it only identifies how this particular type of chronic pain might start. Crucially, it identifies a specific pathway for a specific type of chronic pain. Beyond knowing how to prevent the onset of this type of chronic pain, this is also important because stratifying pain makes it a lot easier to develop specific treatments. Think of it like this: years ago, we thought breast cancer was one kind of cancer, but now we know it's at least ten different types and treatments vary depending on the specific type you have, as they focus on different things. It works so much better. Imagine if, with chronic pain, instead of your doctor giving you the options of paracetamol, anti-inflammatories or opioids and hoping for the best, you were able to find out what type of chronic pain you had and then treat it accordingly? So chronic pain would be more of an umbrella term or starting point.

Why should we care how researchers classify chronic pain? A specific mechanism and a specific pathway are crucial for designing therapies. 'It's only by knowing what to design it against that you can design it,' Dr Bewick says. 'This is why I'm so excited about what we've identified.' It took nearly 30 years for them to identify this GluK2 glutamate receptor. 'And now, putting it together with the work Professor Chen's spent 25 or more years working on ASICs, that makes our work really useful. Which is really, really exciting.' This might be the start of understanding what could be a target for this type of chronic pain.

Professor Chen says, 'I think this is a very unique pathway, and we're really excited about that. This is a totally new direction for chronic pain drug development. There's no doubt about that. And there are several different targets we can focus on.' This is because they know so much about this system, having studied it for so many years.

But the really big question is: how hard is it going to be to turn this breakthrough into a new treatment? He tells me about a treatment called prolotherapy. One example of this therapy is something called PRP therapy – platelet-rich plasma therapy – that's widely used in Asia and the United States. Platelets are important in blood clot formation, immunity, inflammation and wound healing, among other things. Platelet-rich plasma comes from your own blood, and healthcare providers process your blood to concentrate the number of platelets in the plasma and then inject it back into your body. PRP treatment appears to reduce pain and improve function in patients with musculoskeletal pain that has already developed.

PRP contains growth factors that enhance the release of inflammatory mediators and modulators that exert anti-inflammatory and pain-killing effects. It counteracts the inflammatory cascade and has been shown to induce the release of some things that might sound familiar from the meds used to treat certain conditions, for example drugs used to that treat arthritis like Humira, Flurbiprofen and Etoricoxib. It's a pretty expensive therapy, though, and Professor Chen says there are less expensive prolotherapy versions that use 5 to 20 per cent glucose instead, but which have very similar effects to PRP. It's been used in the USA and Taiwan in rehabilitation medicine for a long time now.

One of the pathways these researchers want to use for a druggable target has been used accidentally by rehabilitation medicine for more than 50 years. The prolotherapy injection described above – those injections of glucose into the muscle – can trigger the muscle fibre to release something called Substance P. Substance P is a peptide molecule which acts in the CNS as a neurotransmitter – it lives in part of the brain that's important for affecting behaviour and the neurochemical response to stress. It's also involved in nociceptive (pain) pathways, and is there at sites of inflammation, as inflammation can enhance its expression.

When noxious stimuli occur, pain-sensing fibres send electrical signals along their nerves from the periphery to the central connections in the spinal cord and release Substance P. This can amplify pain signals by sensitising other nerve cells nearby. These signals are then used to tell the CNS that there's a painful stimulus in the periphery.

The pain-sensing fibres can also secrete Substance P in the periphery, where it causes inflammation and also makes the area around it more sensitive. This is how you get a rash and pain during inflammation.

So, if it were Deliveroo: The noxious stimulation is like you placing your order, Substance P is your driver and he goes to pick up your food. He goes from the restaurant to your place, and releases your food. When that's done, you get a notification that the food – or painful stimulus – has been delivered.

'But,' Professor Chen tells me. 'There's one exception, and it's inside muscle.' When prolotherapy injects glucose into muscle, it causes substance P to be released from the acid-sensing nerve fibres that cause sng. This process happens, but in this case it doesn't cause neurogenic inflammation in the muscle. Instead, as they identified in their paper in 2022, Substance P here actually opens an important potassium channel which silences the proprioceptive neurons, actually keeping them from firing. 'That's how this prolotherapy, especially treatments with high concentrations of glucose, have their pain-relief mechanism,' Professor Chen says.

STOPPING INFLAMMATION AND REPAIRING IT TOO 13

I first read about Professor Pere Santamaria, Cumming School of Medicine, Department of Microbiology at the University of Calgary, in a *Nature* article that was absolutely astonishing. That idea I had about CAR T-cell therapy quickly faded because what Professor Santamaria is doing is so much more exciting. CAR T-cell therapy would reboot my immune system, but Professor Santamaria's new treatment – if it works in people as it does in mouse models – will target the specific bit of the immune system that's causing the unwanted inflammation and stop it. But it gets even better: not only will it stop this unwanted inflammation, it will reverse it.

'If you had asked me twenty years ago whether I thought it would be possible to actually suppress immunity in a disease-specific manner, without compromising normal immunity, I would have said no,' Professor Santamaria says. 'I didn't know how it could be done. If you ask me the same question today, and I had not made this discovery, I would answer exactly the same way. I would say no. I don't think it's possible.'

Twenty years ago, he was doing research on autoimmunity 'simply because that's the area I was interested in and was doing curiosity-driven research. I wanted to understand mechanisms of these diseases,' he says, so he could potentially one day identify targets for therapeutic intervention. In the course of this research, they discovered a new class of drugs, 'completely by serendipity. Because I was using these compounds for imaging experiments. I was interested in imaging inflammation. We wanted to be able to measure inflammation of a tissue affected by an autoimmune disease. In this case it was type 1 diabetes using MRI.'

Professor Santamaria developed something similar to the tracer you might use/experience in a PET scan and used it to track the migration (from the bloodstream into the pancreas) of a specific type of immune cell that participates in the immune response that causes diabetes. It occurred to him that, based on what was known about the immune system at the time, 'I might be able to induce tolerance using these compounds.' As in, he could essentially tell the immune system to calm down and chill out. And if he could do that, then he might make a dent on the immune response. 'Not a significant dent, but a dent nonetheless,' he says.

He did the experiments, 'and the results were very, very weird, very counterintuitive. The animals were not developing disease, which means that the compounds were protecting them from disease, but they carried more immune cells capable of recognising the insulin-producing cells of the pancreas in their bodies.'

Professor Santamaria almost 'swept the idea under the carpet, because it didn't make any sense to me, but I let it sit for a few days,' he says. He decided to see, if he made enough assumptions, if he could find a way of explaining his results: 'I realised that if these results were true and I could understand them, then I might be able to discover something important. That I could help people who have autoimmune disease, and that is the objective of our work, right? The objective of our work is not to publish papers and get grants; the objective of our work is to actually make discoveries that will have a meaningful impact on people's lives. So I decided to continue working on that.'

Thank goodness he did. He had no idea how this tracer was working, but it was doing something, and at the expense of everything else he was doing in his lab, he decided to try to figure out how and why this tracer worked. Because he felt it was important and he was curious. This way of working 'is different from what happens when somebody has an idea and says, "OK, I have a pathway in the immune system," for example, "and if I target this step and that other step, I might be able to do something. So I'll design a drug that will target this step." And so you design a drug that targets that step. In my case, it was just the opposite. I have this drug in my hands, that I had no idea how it was working.'

Excitedly, I suggest he's accidentally invented a cure. 'I don't want to call it a cure, because until we know for sure that it works, I think it's dangerous. It was serendipity,' he says. 'But now we know exactly how it works and the mechanisms are fascinating. You could not have predicted it even today, even with everything we know, nobody could have ever designed this drug with current knowledge. Impossible,' he says.

It's taken them twenty years to work it out, going step by step. These drugs are nanoparticles that are decorated with a 'bait' (antigen) for immune cells that participate in specific autoimmune diseases. They're injected intravenously and quickly eliminated by scavengers like the liver macrophages as well as other macrophages (white blood cells), that gobble the nanoparticles up and then dispose of them. But there's a significant number of these nanoparticles that land on the surface of a particular cell type that exists in the spleen, and also in lymph nodes. This type of cell organises what's called a germinal centre reaction, which is the reaction that happens when you get a viral or bacterial vaccine, which essentially exposes fragments of specific pathogens to your immune system so that your immune system can respond very quickly and fight the pathogen when it infects you.

What Professor Santamaria couldn't have predicted was that the 'bait'-coated nanoparticles were just landing on the cell membrane of that cell type but weren't getting internalised. What normally happens is that macrophages eat them and destroy them and digest them. 'But there they were sitting on the surface, as imaged with electron microscopy,' he says.

The nanoparticles selectively reprogrammed a specific type of white blood cell that lives in the same neighbourhood as the cells that landed the nanoparticles. When these white blood cells bite the 'bait' on the nanoparticles, they divide vigorously and acquire the ability to suppress inflammation – they become a small army of protective, yet disease-specific, white blood cells that are capable of disbanding the much larger army of white blood cells that are inflaming the tissues, telling them to go away. This stops inflammation in the organ that is being attacked.

'These protective white blood cells can only suppress inflammation of the tissues that express the "bait". That is, they're only activated when they recognise the antigen local at that site. They basically make all the inflammatory cells go away. In turn, this short circuits the tissue destruction that leads to the self-perpetuating immune response that sustains a chronic autoimmune disease,' he says. Eventually, all the inflammation is gone, and that's when the really exciting thing happens: reversal of the disease.

'Natural evolution has equipped the immune system with cells that can not only suppress immune responses, but also repair the damage caused by such immune responses,' he says. The white blood cells that are reprogrammed by our 'bait'-coated nanoparticles also acquire this property. For example, in diseases like multiple sclerosis (MS), the myelin sheaths are damaged, so I wonder if this new drug might also help people with MS? Could it reverse the damage there?

'Yeah,' he says. 'We see that in mice. The treatment is not just clearing the inflammation, but is also promoting some tissue repair. Now, we don't know if this will also happen in humans with MS or other autoimmune diseases, but certainly what we're seeing in mouse models is very effective. We're hopeful that this is going to work very well in humans too, but we still don't know.' Yet.

Most of Professor Santamaria's work has been on type 1 diabetes, but early on, when he'd made this discovery, he started to branch out, asking the question of 'whether or not what I was seeing in models of diabetes would also occur in models of other autoimmune diseases'.

The drugs they've created are called Navacims and are being developed by Parvus Therapeutics, founded by Professor Santamaria. The first disease that Parvus Therapeutics is working on treating is called primary biliary cholangitis (or primary biliary cirrhosis), which is a type of liver disease that gets worse over time and without treatment leads to liver failure. Right now, they're in Phase I trials – first in human safety trials. Their objective is to demonstrate safety and proof of mechanism in humans. And once they can show that this drug is safe and the mechanism works in humans ... things get even more exciting. 'We have designed other drug candidates for a pipeline of disease indications, inflammatory bowel disease being next,' Professor Santamaria says.

The drug and the way it works should be applicable to a broad range of autoimmune diseases, as is the case in mice, but there are a lot of hurdles to get through first, and Professor Santamaria is careful to caution my excitement: 'All of this is enormously expensive. Drug development is extremely challenging because going from basic academic research and translating that into a drug requires resources and skill sets that are beyond what's available at academic institutions.' For example, drug development needs engineers to make it possible to produce the drug safely and at scale. If any of you take biologics at home, the little injection pen you use was created by an engineer. 'It's one thing to make a little bit of the drug for mouse studies. But it's quite another thing to treat humans. You have to make kilograms of the drug and it has to be cost effective. All of these considerations are super important and that's very challenging to do. You need to understand how to do regulatory documentation, how to organise and execute clinical trials. It costs an enormous amount of money,' he says. 'What I'm saying is, we've luckily overcome the many obstacles in front of us from the time we made the discovery to now, but there is still a lot of work ahead of us. Fortunately, we are in clinical trials now and we should be able to find out soon, and so far so good.'

Professor Santamaria wants to move swiftly. 'Once you get to the clinic, time is of the essence. I would want to go as fast as we possibly can, obviously.' He reminds me how long things take, and about what a tricky thing it is to be an academic and be asked when the new drug is going to be ready. 'You know, sometimes someone says, "Oh, it'll be in the clinic in five years."' He shakes his head. As an example, take what happened with monoclonal antibodies. They're used to treat lots of diseases like cancer, arthritis and IBD. So, César Milstein first started working on the research that would lead to the discovery of monoclonal antibodies in the 1960s. The first monoclonal antibody was produced by Milstein and Gorges Köhler in 1975. In 1986, Orthoclone became the first monoclonal antibody approved by the FDA. It wasn't until the

1990s that these drugs experienced significant growth. That's a good 30 years. The point, though, is that it takes time to learn how to make the drug and optimise it for delivery. It's a lot easier to make another antibody, because we already know how to make those, but Professor Santamaria is making an entirely new drug. This requires a new process.

'Imagine if you discover another technique or another technology,' he says. 'You need to learn everything from scratch. You need to learn how to make it, how to scale the drug up. You run into all kinds of problems. You have to re-engineer molecules. And these things, they're not fast, and they're super expensive.' The pressure he's under to do this for all of us is clear. 'Failure is the rule of the day,' he says. He's not being pessimistic; this is how scientific discovery works. A negative result, while obviously disappointing, is still useful information. 'What I've experienced across these two decades is two steps forward and one step backwards; it's very challenging and difficult,' he says. But the fact that Parvus Therapeutics is in clinical trials means that things are moving in the right direction.

Professor Santamaria tells me that if someone had told him how challenging all of this was going to be, he wouldn't have believed them, that he wouldn't have understood: 'But having lived through it and knowing what kind of problems you run into – the challenge of raising money with investors when there is a scepticism because it sounds too good to be true or because at that time we didn't understand the mechanism. And we didn't know how many diseases we would be able to target and so on so forth.' It was an uphill battle. Especially because as academics and scientists, there were so many other things they didn't know about that were outside their expertise – he'd never developed a drug before, he's not a serial entrepreneur so he didn't know how to raise funds in that space, or even how best to communicate his ideas to investors. The entire process has been a learning curve fraught with challenges. But regardless of this, he's convinced that the new drug will address an important unmet need in the treatment of autoimmune disease.

The other thing he's really keen to talk about is how much scientists don't know, and I couldn't be more grateful to him for his honesty about this. So often it feels like we think and expect doctors and scientists to know the answers to ALL our problems, but they simply don't: 'We know a lot less than there is to know. We know a fraction of what there is to know, and in my case I was lucky enough to run into this sort of serendipitous observation. And I took the risk to explore it. But the fact that twenty years later there's nothing that works better than this, that tells you something, doesn't it?' It certainly does.

'When I look back, there's been a lot of frustration and pain over the years. I haven't had any fun. But I pinch myself because we're getting closer to maybe being able to help people. I think that's my most important contribution – it's our goal. As scientists our ultimate goal is to provide solutions to people's health problems. Most of the time we fail. Other times we generate information that others can use to be successful. But that's our objective.'

How does it feel for him knowing how many people his work has the potential to help?

'I'm happy that I made that decision to go ahead with this research and that there is the opportunity to test it. If it so happens that we're right that the drugs are safe, and that they operate the way we know they're operating in animals and they treat people the same way, then I will feel enormous pleasure of having been able to help people,' he says.

THE END

It's a Friday before the late May bank holiday and I am in agony – it's been building for a couple of days, but now it's intolerable. My manager at work, who is lovely and understanding, has told me to go to bed and not come to a meeting. The pain is in a few old favourite spots and a couple of new ones, but it's also more urgent and all encompassing. I'm used to it turning up and staying put in my ribs, but today it's got other ideas and sets out on an adventure around my midsection. I hurt – a lot – from my neck to my hips, so I dutifully fill out my GP's e-consult form and a few hours later am told that I could be seen in four weeks' time. Not great, but I'm too tired and feel too awful to argue. Besides, I understand that the NHS is in bad shape at the moment, and I have to trust that the doctor who's triaged my request has assessed the situation properly.

But I need to do something to shift the pain because it really is all-consuming. My personal chronic pain pharmacy hasn't helped, so I decide to visit the pharmacist and see if she has any bright ideas. I ask my partner to come with me because that seems sensible, though what he'll be able to do isn't immediately obvious. But I am not feeling right and sometimes you need someone. Just in case.

I walk – uphill – bent over, holding my tummy as if that might help, and I keep asking my partner to slow down, which is completely out of character. Normally it's the other way around and I'm charging ahead, barely even noticing that we're going uphill. We go into the pharmacy and the pharmacist smiles in recognition and I raise my hand to greet her, and even that feels like too much. I gesture to where it hurts and ask what she thinks it might be or what might help.

What she thinks is that I need to be seen by the GP, urgently.

Eventually, around four in the afternoon, the GP phones and I describe my symptoms – pain in the rib cage, pain down both sides, pain in my stomach. I feel breathless, winded. The GP says I should come and see her, so, at four-thirty on a Friday before a bank holiday, I drag myself back up the hill. I'm out of breath when I get there, which is worrying considering that I am generally – diseases aside – fairly fit.

As I wait to be seen I think about how this book turned out. I started out trying to find a cellular target to use in a trial on AS with CAR T-cell therapy, and I didn't find it. I really did picture this ending differently – and I know it was a long shot, but still, long shots work out sometimes, right? And I don't even think it's that much of a long shot – given everyone I've met in the course of writing this book – to think that new treatments are on their way. Who's it going to be? Professor Lee at the Crick, finding a way to use a different cancer drug to treat inflammation? Professor Santamaria in Calgary with his nano-medicines? Or maybe Professor Noel and her colleagues will develop a way for us to re-wire our brains. Maybe all those things and more will happen.

But we're not there now and I wish we were, because I'm really impatient. Or maybe it's more accurate to say I've been waiting my whole life for things to get better. I'm ready. I don't want to wait any longer. I think back to what Professor Leandro told me – that we should be grateful for the biologics we have and that I take. These weren't available when I was first diagnosed and they're a really good treatment option – they change people's lives for the better.

To be a patient, you need a lot of patience. That word was first used sometime in the first half of the twelfth century to mean tolerant; by the second half of the fourteenth century a new sense was added: that of enduring hardship without complaint. Here's another part of the definition: Able to continue a course of action without being daunted by difficulties or hindrances; persevering, diligent; painstaking. That applies as much to the people who are sick as it does to the researchers we've heard from: they're enduring a sort of hardship when results don't work out the way they've expecting, they're persevering, they're diligent and they're certainly continuing a course of action without being daunted. I like that we have those qualities in common. That makes me feel like we really are on the same team.

And I know we are, and I know they want these new treatments to get to us faster because they want to help – that's the whole reason behind their research. They want to make the lives of people like us – people with chronic pain – better.

When I started this project I was joking with my sister, who also has AS. Imagine, I said, imagine if I can find a cellular target, and then also a few million pounds, and we start a clinical trial, and I can be part of it, and we do the CAR T-cell therapy, and it actually works, and then I will be well. She flat out laughed at me. Not the idea of finding the right target and starting a clinical trial – no – she laughed at the absurdity of being well. And that's what so many of the people who live with chronic pain told me. Not one of them could remember what it was like to not be in pain, and none of them could imagine what it would be like to be well again. I don't think that's just a failure of our imaginations – chronic pain changes who and how you are, as all experiences do, but in a world that's constantly changing, where we switch jobs and move house and break up and get together with new people all the time, chronic pain is one of those rare constants. It's always there. Even if it's not being super loud, you know it's there, lurking in the background.

I'm called in to see the GP around five o'clock. She examines me and says, apologetically, that she doesn't know what's wrong but that it seems like I'm suffering from some kind of all-over myalgia. She gives me some codeine, books me for blood tests, and sends me on my way. I try to pass on the codeine, because it's not great for Crohn's, but she reminds me it is the weekend and I might need a little help to get through it. I take the script.

And I take the codeine, which rather predictably makes me feel nauseous and doesn't really help. After a mostly sleepless night, I get out of bed and go down a weird rabbit hole on the internet. Maybe my pain is a Crohn's flare, so I ditch the high-fibre diet in favour of a soft white foods minibreak, and that seems to help enough for me to function.

When my blood tests came back, they showed that I was really low in iron, again, still, and that some other things were positive when they should have been negative – further testing was needed.

There's every chance I'm fine. Unfortunately, my mission to find a target for CAR T-cell therapy to treat my AS has been a bust. But it hasn't been for naught because I've learned a lot – new ideas for how I might retrain my brain and how the changes menopause brings with it might also be contributing to an increase in pain. Even the stuff I've learned that doesn't directly impact me just yet – Professor Santamaria's work, Dr Loggia's, Professor Price's, Dr Johnston's – it reminds me that even though there are millions of us suffering with pain, there are also so many researchers out there trying to help. We aren't being left on our own to suffer; people are there, thinking, researching, understanding, and it'll all come to something. Eventually.

We just need to be a little more patient.

Oh, and just one more thing: months have passed since this strange outburst from my body, and it turns out I was developing antibodies to my infusion. So I won't be seeing

Jolly again anytime soon. I'll be trying new medications – or, as I like to call it, playing biologic bingo – instead.

The researchers listed below are the heroes of this book and I cannot thank them enough for their time and their hard work.

Name	Title	Institution
Amanda Williams	Professor of Clinical Health Psychology	UCL
Simon Beggs	Associate Professor, Developmental Neuroscience	UCL
Maria Leandro	Associate Professor, Consultant Rheumatologist	UCL and UCLH
Chris Eccleston	Professor, Department for Health, Centre for Pain Research	University of Bath
Melanie Noel	Professor of Clinical Psychology	University of Calgary
Richelle Mychasiuk	Professor, Department of Neuroscience	University of Sydney
Fiona Watt	Clinical Associate Professor in Rheumatology, UKRI Future Leaders Fellow	Imperial College London
Parsad Shirvalkar	Associate Professor, Anaesthesia	University of California, San Francisco
Marco Loggia	Professor of Radiology, Associate Professor of Anaesthesia, Co-Director, Center for Integrative Pain NeuroImaging	Harvard Medical School

Name	Title	Institution
Theodore Price	Ashbel Smith Professor, Department of Neuroscience	The University of Texas at Dallas
James Lee	Clinician Scientist Group Leader, Genetic Mechanisms of Disease Laboratory Consultant Gastroenterologist (Royal Free)	The Francis Crick Institute
Paul Wordsworth	Professor of Rheumatology, Nuffield Department of Orthopaedics, Rheumatology and Musculoskeletal Sciences;	University of Oxford
Keira Johnston	Associate Research Scientist of Psychiatry	Yale School of Medicine
Massieh Moyadei	Associate Professor, Faculty of Dentistry	University of Toronto
David Seminowicz	Professor, Medical Biophysics[; Robarts Research Institute	University of Western Ontario
Blair Smith	Professor, Chair of Population Health Science	University of Dundee
Stefan Siebert	Professor of Inflammation Medicine and Rheumatology	University of Glasgow
Guy Bewick	Senior Lecturer, Institute of Medical Sciences	University of Aberdeen
Chih-Cheng Chen	Distinguished Research Fellow, Institute of Biomedical Sciences	Academic Sinica, Taiwan
David Andersson	Professor of Neuroscience	King's College London

Name	Title	Institution
Jeffrey Mogil	Professor, Canada Research Chair in Genetics of Pain	McGill University
Pere Santamaria	Professor, Department of Microbiology Immunity and Infestion	University of Calgary
Raj Sengupta	Professor Consultant Rheumatologist	University of Bath Royal National Hospital for Rheumatic Diseases

ACKNOWLEDGEMENTS

There are many people whose help was invaluable to me while I was writing this book:

The team at Icon – Connor Stait, Elle-Jay Christodoulou, Amelia Kemmer and Steve Burdett – who have all worked tirelessly to help shepherd the book along.

Dr Krista Schleicher for her help with molecular genetics.

The people like me who live with chronic pain and kindly shared their stories with me – thank you.

The Society of Authors for giving me a grant to work on this project.

My agent, Anna Pallai, who helped me to shape this idea into something I'm very proud of.

And, of course, my partner, Connor Walsh, who took on the lion's share of housework and life admin so I could work on this – and who is always ready to help do whatever he can to ease my aches and pains.

INDEX

Aberdeen, University of 231
abuse 6, 40, 41, 42, 53, 62
Academia Sinica, Taiwan 231
acid-sensing ion channels (ASICs) 235–6, 238
ADHD 177–8
Advanced Pain Discovery Platform 155
adverse childhood experiences (ACEs) 37, 41–3, 201
alpha brain waves 177–80
ALS 115
Alzheimer's disease 112, 185
American Association of Medical Colleges 87
amitriptyline 76
amygdala 64, 69–70
anaesthesia 46, 66–7, 118, 192
Andersson, Professor David 228–31
animal models 2, 6, 56, 63–4, 67, 70–1, 73, 78–80, 92, 95–6, 98, 106–7, 112, 119–21, 164, 217–24, 228–9, 233, 236–7, 243, 247–9
ankylosing spondylitis (AS) x–xi, 9–11, 12, 16, 24–5, 43–5, 65, 91, 108, 137, 139–41, 143–4, 145, 147, 148–9, 151, 153–5, 195, 201, 210–13, 215, 253–6
antibiotics 136, 137
antibodies 19–20, 24, 91, 149, 211–12, 228–31, 249
anti-inflammatories xii, 55, 72, 75, 100, 238, 239
antiracism 191
anti-TNF 24–5, 148; *see also* Tumour Necrosis Factor alpha blocker
anxiety 2, 39, 46, 61, 62, 68–70, 80, 91, 185
arthritis x–xi, 7, 24, 35, 99, 102, 105, 106, 135, 147, 148, 153, 197, 208, 213, 219
ASICs *see* acid-sensing ion channels
assay 217, 219–20, 221, 223
attention 34, 51, 77, 168–9, 176
Austin, Dr Jehannine (J9) 161–2
autoantibodies 17, 19, 24, 229, 230

autoimmune disease x, 12, 19, 50, 55, 98, 105–8, 134–43, 230–1, 244–8, 251
autoimmunity 106, 163, 244

B cells 17–24, 141, 210
babies 35, 46–7, 55–6, 63–4, 66–7, 691–7, 79
baclofen xii
bacterial infection 135–7
Banks, Dr Robert 233–4
Bath, University of 27, 29
Bath Pain Centre 29
B-cell depletion therapy *see* rituximab
Beggs, Dr Simon 7, 65–74, 75, 78, 79–80
bereavement 188
Bewick, Dr Guy 231–8
biases 51, 92–4, 96–7, 176, 200
biologics 50, 91, 100–1, 104, 123, 127–8, 142–3, 147–8, 150, 154, 189, 196, 197, 200, 211–13, 229–30, 249, 255, 257–8
biomarker 178–9, 209
bladder pain 127
body image 171–2, 173–6
brain efficiencies 37
brain stimulation 81–4
brain waves 177
Brewerton, Professor Derek 139–40
British Columbia (Canada), University of 161

calcitonin gene-related peptide *see* CGRP
calcium 101
Calgary, University of 38, 243
California, University of 41, 81, 84, 127
cancer xii, 12, 17, 28, 41, 91, 112, 117–18, 126–8, 150, 171, 193, 203–4, 215, 238
Cancer Research UK 134
cancer.org 13
cannabinoids 169
capsaicin 84
CAR (chimeric antigen receptor) 12
CAR T-cell therapy 12–14, 16, 17–24, 50, 128, 148–9, 210, 243, 254, 256, 257
CAR T cells 12–13, 17–18, 22–3, 149
cardiac dysrhythmia 163
catastrophic thinking 189–91
CBC (Canada) 168
CBT *see* cognitive behavioural therapy
cell cycle neuroplasticity 163
cells xiv, 12–13, 17–25, 59, 64, 71, 81, 84, 92, 95, 112, 114, 118–19, 121–2, 126, 128, 134–5, 139, 141–3, 147–9, 150, 152, 163, 164, 210, 228, 230, 233–5, 240, 244–7
central nervous system (CNS) 5, 70, 80, 111, 115–16, 234, 240
CGRP (calcitonin gene-related peptide) 95
Charon, Rita 49–50
chemotherapy 2, 203
Chen, Professor Chih-Cheng 231–2, 235–41
Child Health, Institute of 65
childbirth xi, 55, 96, 87
childhood experiences 36–42, 46–7, 54–6, 79–80, 124, 170, 201
children 28, 33, 36–7, 38–43, 46–7, 54–6, 60, 62–5, 66–8, 69–70, 79–80, 94, 97, 137, 167, 170, 177–8, 201, 202

chimeric antigen
receptor *see* CAR
cholangitis, primary biliary 248
cholangitis, primary
sclerosing 145
chromosome 21 144
clinical trials 14–16, 17–19, 20–2, 72–7, 81, 84, 96, 121–2, 129, 145, 149, 151, 181, 219, 224–5, 230, 248–50, 256
Cochrane Group 72
codeine xii, 91, 206, 256–7
cognition 34–5, 180, 182
cognitive behavioural therapy (CBT) 196
colitis *see* inflammatory bowel disease
Columbia University, New York 49
community 42–3, 48–9, 53
complex disease 161
complex disease trait 159–62
complex regional pain syndrome (CRPS) 59, 174, 175, 195, 228
connective tissues 101, 103–4
connectivity map 164
cortisol 55
costochondritis xi
Craig, Kenneth 2
Crick, Francis 133
Crohn's disease x, 134, 138, 148, 197, 204, 210, 211, 256–7
see also inflammatory bowel disease
Culture of Pain, The 168
cytokine release storms 22, 23
cytokine release syndrome (CRS) 13
cytokines 13, 54–5, 100, 122, 142, 163, 196
Darwin, Charles 159
depression 5, 39, 40, 41, 42, 46, 59, 62, 68, 81, 91, 94, 113, 161, 162, 171–2, 185, 189, 209
diabetes 4, 119–20, 134, 138, 143, 244, 248
diabetic peripheral neuropathy *see* pain: peripheral neuropathy
diet *see* nutrition
disability-adjusted life years (DALY) 195
Disease Control, Centers for (USA) 202
DNA 60, 84, 125, 134, 135–6, 145–6, 159, 162
dorsal root
ganglia (DRG) 117–19
drug companies *see*
pharmaceutical companies
Dundee, University of 187
Durham University 233
dyspareunia 164

Eccleston, Professor Chris 27–33, 94
Edwards, Professor Jonathan 19, 20
EEG (electroencephalogram) 177, 178
empathy 43, 45, 46–8, 49, 50, 65, 69, 77, 131, 197
endometriosis 164, 201
Engel, George 195
environmental factor/trigger 6, 30, 34, 40, 80, 101, 126, 134, 136–8, 140, 160–1, 222
EPICure UK cohort 69
epidemiology 80, 103, 187, 209
epigenetics 40, 60, 63
Epstein Barr virus 138

Etoricoxib 239
evolution 33, 62, 134–6, 169, 247
exercise 30, 101, 204–6

Farmer, Dr Melissa 220
fatigue 5, 18, 19, 22, 68, 76, 163, 209
feedback loop 169, 176, 233
Felitti, Dr Vincent J. 41
female health gap 92–3
fibromyalgia 65, 105, 108, 114, 164, 195, 197, 229–31, 232
fluconazole 220
Flurbiprofen 239
Francis Crick Institute (the Crick) 133, 144
funding 15, 75, 78, 149, 155, 156–7, 181, 215, 249–51

GABA 169
gastrointestinal infection (GI) 138
gender equity 190–1
gender inequality *see* pain: sex-differences
gene desert 144, 146, 152
generational transmission 38
genes 12, 60–3, 84, 92, 95, 118–19, 122, 125, 134–5, 143–7, 159–65, 199, 201
  see also sequencing *and* next-generation sequencing
  COL11A1 125
  ETS2 134–5, 144–5, 147, 149–54
  GDF5 125
  HLA-B27 139–42, 143
  HLA-DRB1 125
  IL-23 142–3, 144
  NOD2 138
  P2X7 125
  RUNX3 143
  TNF 125
  TRPV1 125
genetics 17, 40, 54, 115–6, 120, 127, 133–5, 139–54, 159–65, 168, 199, 205
genome-wide association studies (GWAS) 140, 143–4, 161–2, 164
genomics 135, 140–1, 144
genotype 217–18
germinal centre reaction 246
Glasgow, University of 208
glial cells 112, 114
GluK2 235, 238
glutamate 234–8
Great Ormond Street Institute of Child Health (UCL) 7, 65–6
grief 2, 188
Guardian 12
Gulf War Syndrome 114
gut microbiome 137, 142
GWAS *see* genome-wide association studies

Harvard Medical School 76
HEAL initiative 129
HIV 212
hope 12, 131, 154, 185
hormones 55, 63, 71, 88, 98–108
HRT (hormone replacement therapy) 99, 101, 102, 103–4, 108–9
Humira 239
Huntington's disease 115, 159–60
Hussein, Dr 43
hyper-responsive/hyper-reactive/hypersensitive 54, 68

IASP see International Association for the Study of Pain
IBD *see* inflammatory bowel disease
ICOS 128
IL-17 (cytokine) 142–3
IL-17 blockers 91
IL6 101
immune cells 70, 95, 114–15, 121, 143, 230, 244, 246–7
immune effector cell-associated neurotoxicity syndrome (ICANS) 23
immune system x, 12–13, 18–23, 54, 55–6, 61, 68–70, 78–80, 95, 100, 117, 121, 128, 134–5, 136, 141, 147, 155, 171, 200, 208, 229, 243–7
immunology neuropsychiatrist 209
Imperial College London 99, 134
inflammatory bowel disease (IBD) 134, 137–8, 143, 144–7, 149, 150, 152–4, 195, 248 *see also* Crohn's disease
inflammatory disease x, 24, 98, 135, 145, 150–1, 170–1, 196, 208–9, 211, 219
inflammatory macrophage *see* macrophages
interleukins 211
International Association for the Study of Pain (IASP) 4, 27, 68, 88–9, 193
International Classification of Diseases (ICD) 194–5
interstitial cystitis 164
ion channel proteins 228
iPain 125
isolation 52–3, 68

JAK inhibitors 211
Johnston, Dr Keira 159–65
Journal of Pain, The 190
Journavx 77
Julius, Professor David 84

Katherine 18–19
Keystone, Dr Edward 32, 44–5, 207
kidney stones xi
King's College London 40, 134, 228
kNOw pain 184
Köhler, Gorges 249
Kringel, Dario 125

LA Times 184
Lancet 5
Leandro, Dr Maria 19–23
Lee, Professor James 133–9, 144–54
leukaemia 12, 22
Lewis, Dr Jenny 175
lidocaine 77
lifestyle 28, 138, 191
Loggia, Professor Marco 111–16
Lötsch, Jörn 125
lupus 12, 17–24, 50, 105, 134, 149, 210
lymphoma 12, 19

Machado, Professor Pedro 14, 16
macrophages 134, 147, 148, 149, 151–2, 246–7
Marmot, Professor Sir Michael 201
Marmot Review (2010) 201
mastectomy 171
maternal separation 63–4
McCall, Davina 109
McGill Pain Index xi

McGill University, Montreal 74, 111, 190
MD Anderson, Texas 117–18
mechanical allodynia 221, 224
Medical Research Council (MRC) 133, 155
MEK inhibitors 150–1
memory 5, 22, 34–5, 29, 40, 113, 185
men 71, 73, 78, 87, 89, 91, 93–7, 106–7, 172, 199, 201–3, 222–3
Mendel, Gregor 159
Mendelian disorder 159
meningitis 112
menopause 88, 98, 99–100, 101–9
methotrexate 211
methylation 60–1
microglia 70–1, 112
migraine 76–7, 91, 95–6, 114, 127, 181–2, 183
Milstein, César 249
mind–body connections 173–5
mindfulness meditation 173, 175, 181
mindfulness-based stress reduction (MBSR) 181–2
Mirage Device, The 173
mirror therapy 173
MNK 121–2
Moayedi, Massieh 167–8, 170–3, 175–6
modulating signals 168
Mogil, Professor Jeffrey 74, 92, 94, 96–7, 217–25, 227–8
mood problems 5
Moore, Pete 208
morphine 203, 206–7
MRI scan 177, 244
mRNA technology 123
multiple sclerosis (MS) 98, 115, 138, 155, 197, 247
multi-sensory integration 173–5
multi-site chronic pain 162
myasthenia gravis 231
Mychasiuk, Professor Richelle 53–62, 95–6, 97–9
myeloma 12

narrative medicine 49–51
National Institute for Medical Research 133
National Institutes of Health (NIH) 72, 78, 127, 129
Nature 126, 243
Nav1.8 inhibitor 127
Navacims 248
neonates 66–8, 69–71, 79–80
nerve damage 4, 23, 204, 219, 228, 247
neurofibromatosis 150
neuroinflammation 111–12
neurologist 81
neurons 31, 57, 64, 70, 84, 111–12, 121–2, 126, 128, 234, 241
neuroscience 40, 71, 83, 111, 122, 170
Neuroscience, Journal of 184
neuroscientist 80, 81, 111
neurotransmitters 91, 240
Newport, Dr Roger 173–5
next-generation sequencing (NGS) 125, 127–8, 129
NHS Confederation 92
nociception 90, 101, 168, 170, 240
nociceptors 4, 6, 101, 122
Noel, Dr Melanie 38–48, 52–3, 63–5, 69, 75, 77, 80, 176, 201
norepinephrine 169

NSAIDs (non-steroidal anti-inflammatories) xii, 72, 91, 147
Nuffield Health 202
numbers-needed-to-treat (NNT) 225
nutrition 56–7, 60–1, 80, 91, 137–8, 160, 257

obesity 28, 120, 137
oestrogen 100–1, 103, 106, 108
oestrous cycle 98
olfactory-mediated analgesia 222–3
oligonucleotide-based technologies 123
opioid misuse 39, 41, 62, 156
opioids 49, 75, 124, 125, 129, 156, 169, 206–7, 238
Origin of Species, On the 159
Orthoclone 249
osteoarthritis 99–105, 107, 125, 171, 173, 174 *see also* arthritis
osteoporosis 101
oxidative stress 163
oxytocin 55

PAIN 29, 90–1, 125, 156
pain
  acceptance of 28, 188–9
  acute 32, 46, 54, 56, 77, 89, 127, 167–9, 188, 192, 224
  age differences 103, 199, 201
  biography 78–9
  biopsychosocial model 195–7
  cancer 91, 127, 168, 171, 193, 203–4
  chronic primary pain 193–5
  classification of 4–6, 193–5
  clinics 182, 188, 194, 202, 215
  and cognition 3, 34, 39, 163, 172, 177, 180, 182, 183
  culture of 38, 46, 48–9, 64–5, 168, 237
  definition of 2–4, 8, 28, 30–1, 193, 198, 203–4, 237–8
  diagnosis 29, 36, 45, 79, 89, 91, 161, 188, 193–4, 198, 202, 204, 213, 230
  education 93, 184, 190–3, 207
  finance 21, 35, 94–5, 109, 153, 155, 194, 197
  imaging 168
  impact of 3, 28–32, 153–6, 203–5
  inflammatory 197
  measuring 7–8, 30, 33–4, 96–7, 112–13, 217, 220–2
  medicine 66, 156, 192–3
  musculoskeletal (MSK) 39, 43, 93, 101–4, 107, 215, 239
  neuropathic 4–5, 6, 28, 77, 84, 95, 118–19, 122, 125, 130–1, 188, 199, 203, 219, 225, 228
  nociceptive 4–5, 6, 90, 101, 122, 168, 170, 240
  nociplastic 5–6, 113, 163–4, 197
  peripheral mechanism of 232 *see also* peripheral nervous system
  peripheral neuropathic 28, 77, 119–20, 130, 219
  physical 3, 30, 33–4, 40, 46, 47, 50, 189, 195
  post-surgical 72–3, 79–80, 116, 127, 130, 171–2, 179, 193, 203–4
  post-traumatic 40, 193

psychological 3, 31, 46, 56, 62, 81, 189, 195, 195
sensitivity to 55, 67–8, 96, 107, 125, 169–70, 179–80, 221, 228–9, 235–7
sex differences 6, 69–72, 78, 87–110, 164, 172, 199, 201–2
sng- 236–7, 240
social aspect of 3, 38–9, 47, 49, 52, 75, 96, 107, 171–2, 195–7, 200
spontaneous 221, 224
statistics 28, 79, 89, 194
symptoms 1, 4, 5–6, 37, 74, 76–7189, 203, 220–2, 229, 254
toolkit 208
variability 167–8, 168–9, 179–80
visceral 84
painkilling system, natural 169–70
paracetamol xiii, 91, 174, 238
Parkinson's disease xi, 155, 185
Parvus Therapeutics 248, 250
pathology 32–3, 39, 227
patient and public involvement *see* PPI
patriarchy 48, 52, 71
peak alpha frequency 178–80
Pennsylvania, University of 127
peripheral nerve stimulation 84
peripheral nervous system (PNS) 4–6, 23, 100, 112, 117, 120–2, 183, 232, 234, 240
pharmaceutical companies 15, 21, 75, 77, 121, 129, 142, 145, 153, 199, 248–9
pharmacist 253–4
pharmacology 72–3, 122, 127, 165, 182, 192, 211
placebo 74–5, 130, 175, 224–5
platelet-rich plasma therapy see PRP
politics 93, 184, 199, 200–1, 213–4
polygenic 140, 143
positive childhood experiences 42, 47–8
PPI (patient and public involvement) 14
pregabalin 225
pregnancy 100
prehabilitation 196
premature ovarian insufficiency 106
prenatal stress 55
Price, Professor Ted 117–23, 128, 130–1
progesterone 100
prolotherapy 239–41
proprioception 233–41
PRP (platelet-rich plasma therapy) therapy 239
psoriasis 134, 211
psoriatic arthritis 24, 153, 208–9, 210, 211, 212
psychology 3, 32–3, 39–8, 56–8, 81, 96, 130, 168, 188–91, 194–5, 200, 201–5, 207–8, 214–5, 227
PTSD 39–41, 42, 46, 56, 162
Pule, Professor Martin 21–2

radiotherapy 203
Remicade 73
research 13–16, 17–22, 87, 93, 106, 151–2, 156, 162–5, 167, 194, 208–10, 217–24, 232–3, 248–50

rheumatoid arthritis 12, 19, 24, 105, 122, 134, 143, 162, 208–9, 210–13, 215
rheumatology xiv, 21, 24, 105, 108–9, 139, 196, 208, 212
Rheumatology, British Society for 139
rituximab 19–21, 24
RNA 61, 125
Royal Free Hospital 154
Royal National Hospital for Rheumatic Diseases, Bath 189, 195, 197, 198
Royal United Hospital, Bath 188

Sahn, James 122
Santamaria, Professor Pere 243–52
Schett, Georg 17
schizophrenia 194
sciatica 77
Science Translational Medicine 76
scleroderma 50
secukinamab 142–4
Seminowicz, Professor David 177–83
senescence 126
Sengupta, Professor Raj 7, 13–14, 16, 189, 195–8, 205
sequencing 60, 118, 124–5, 145–6
serotonin 169
Shirvalkar, Dr Prasad 81–4
Siebert, Stefan 208–14
single nucleotide polymorphisms (SNPs) 141, 162–3
Skoglund, Dr Pontus 135
sleep xiii, 5, 9, 40, 44, 55, 68, 76, 101–3, 113, 114, 163, 177, 182
Smith, Professor Blair 187–9, 193, 198–200, 201–8
smoking 138
SNP heritability 162
SNP *see* single nucleotide polymorphisms
social support 42–3, 54, 64
socioeconomics 43, 80, 93, 200–2, 213–14
somatisation 189
somatosensory nervous system 4, 6, 67, 113, 125–6
South Africa 212
spinal cord 5, 81, 84, 100, 111–12, 113, 117, 121, 169, 183, 232, 240
spinal cord stimulation 84
spondyloarthritis 195, 197, 208
stereotype 94, 107, 171, 202
steroids 18, 72, 147, 212
stickiness 31
stigma 89, 191
stories 44–5, 48, 65
stress 53, 55–8, 60, 61–2, 63–4, 65, 67–8, 76, 80, 137, 161, 168, 170, 181–2, 223, 240
stroke 112, 185
Substance P 240–1
suicide 41, 62–3
Sullivan, Michael 190
surgery 46, 49, 66–7, 69–71, 72–3, 79–80, 92–3, 116, 117, 121, 130–1, 171–2, 203
suzetrigine 127
swimming 32–3, 44, 61, 204–5
Sydney, University of 53

T cells 12, 128, 141–2, 143, 152, 210 *see also* CAR T-cells
testosterone 90, 100, 101

Texas, University of 117
thalamus 112–13, 115
thermal hyperalgesia 221
tinnitus xii
TMD (tempomandibular disorder) 181
TNF alpha 101
TNF-inhibitors 211–12
Toronto 32, 43–4, 168, 207
Toronto, University of 167
Torres, Olga 50
training 93, 109, 153, 184, 190–3, 207
tramadol xii
transcriptome 118–19
translational research/medicine 184, 207, 231
translator protein (TSPO) 112–16
transmagnetic stimulation (TMS) 59–60
trauma 37–42, 46–7, 54–6, 57, 62–5, 90, 107, 124, 161, 181, 212
trigeminal nerve 126
Trump, President 78
trust 47, 49, 51, 94
Tumour Necrosis Factor alpha blocker (TNF) x, xxii; *see also* anti-TNF

UK Biobank 162, 209
ultrasound 82
University College London (UCL) 2, 12–13, 14, 17, 21, 65–6, 94, 134, 201
University College London Hospital 17, 19
uveitis xi

vaccines 123, 246
Vertex 77
Vioxx xii
virtual reality (VR) 59–60, 175
vitamins 9, 61, 101
vulvodynia 164, 201, 220

Wager, Tor 130
Walker, Dr Suellen 66, 69
Watt, Professor Judith 93, 98, 99–110
Wellcome 134
West of England, University of the 175
Western Ontario (Canada), University of 177
whole-body medicine 212
Williams, Professor Amanda 1, 2–3, 94
women 6, 69–72, 78, 87–90, 164, 201, 222
Women and Equalities Committee 89–90
Wordsworth, Professor Paul 139–44
World Health Organization (WHO) 91, 193

Yale School of Medicine 159
yeast infections 220
yoga 173, 176